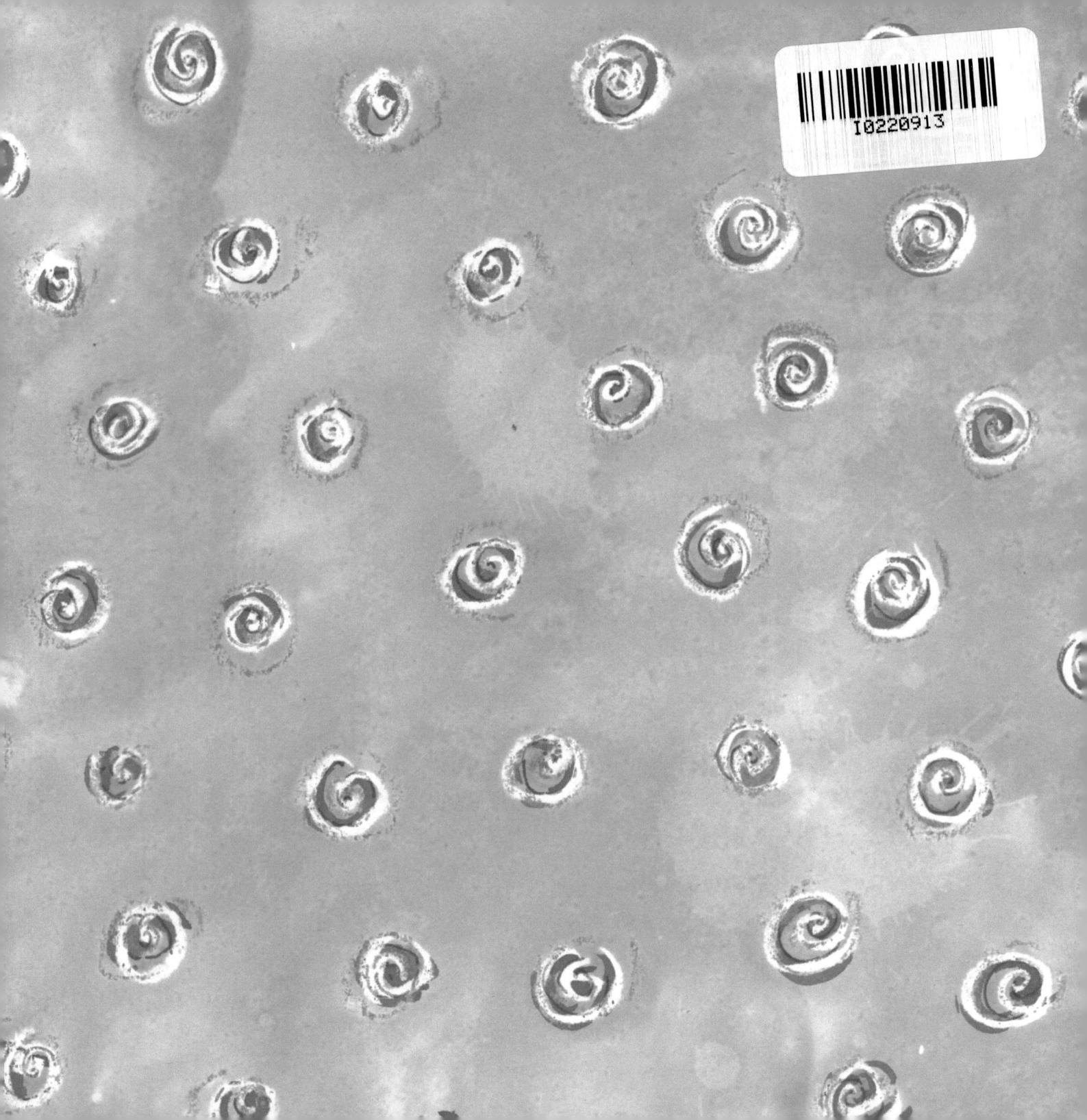

Text copyright © 2011 Carmen Martínez Jover
www.carmenmartinezjover.com
illustrations copyright © 2011 Rosemary Martínez
www.rosemarymartinez.com

A tiny itsy bitsy Gift of Life for Boys
1st edition, November 2011

ISBN 978-607-00-5062-6

Story: Carmen Martinez Jover
Design & illustrations: Rosemary Martinez
Layout: Victor Alfonso Nieto

Personalise books for your kids with your own family names
for boys, girls and twins:
https://books.carmenmartinezjover.com

All rights reserved. This book may not be reproduced,
In whole nor in parts, including illustrations, in any form,
without written permission from the authors.

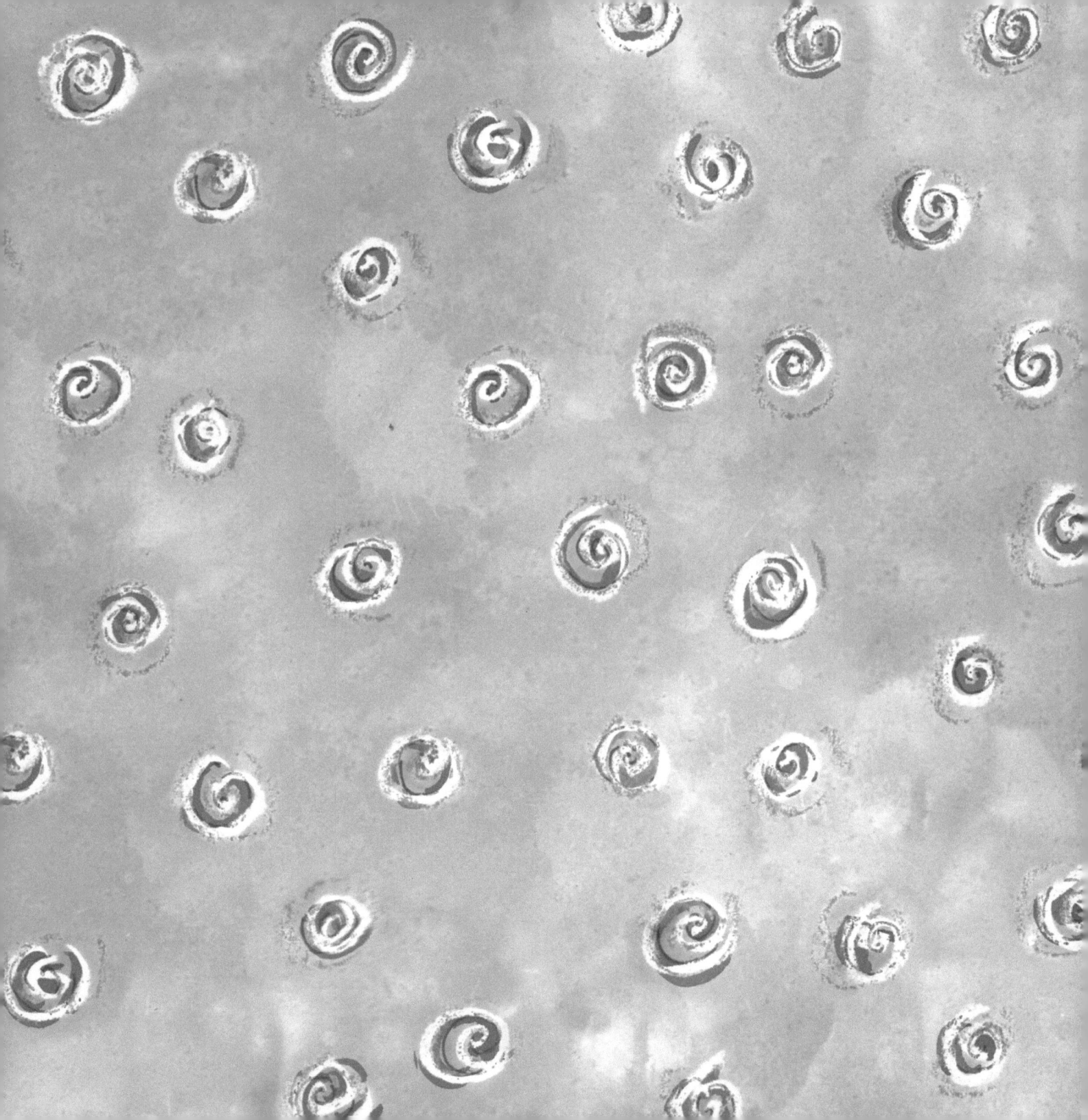

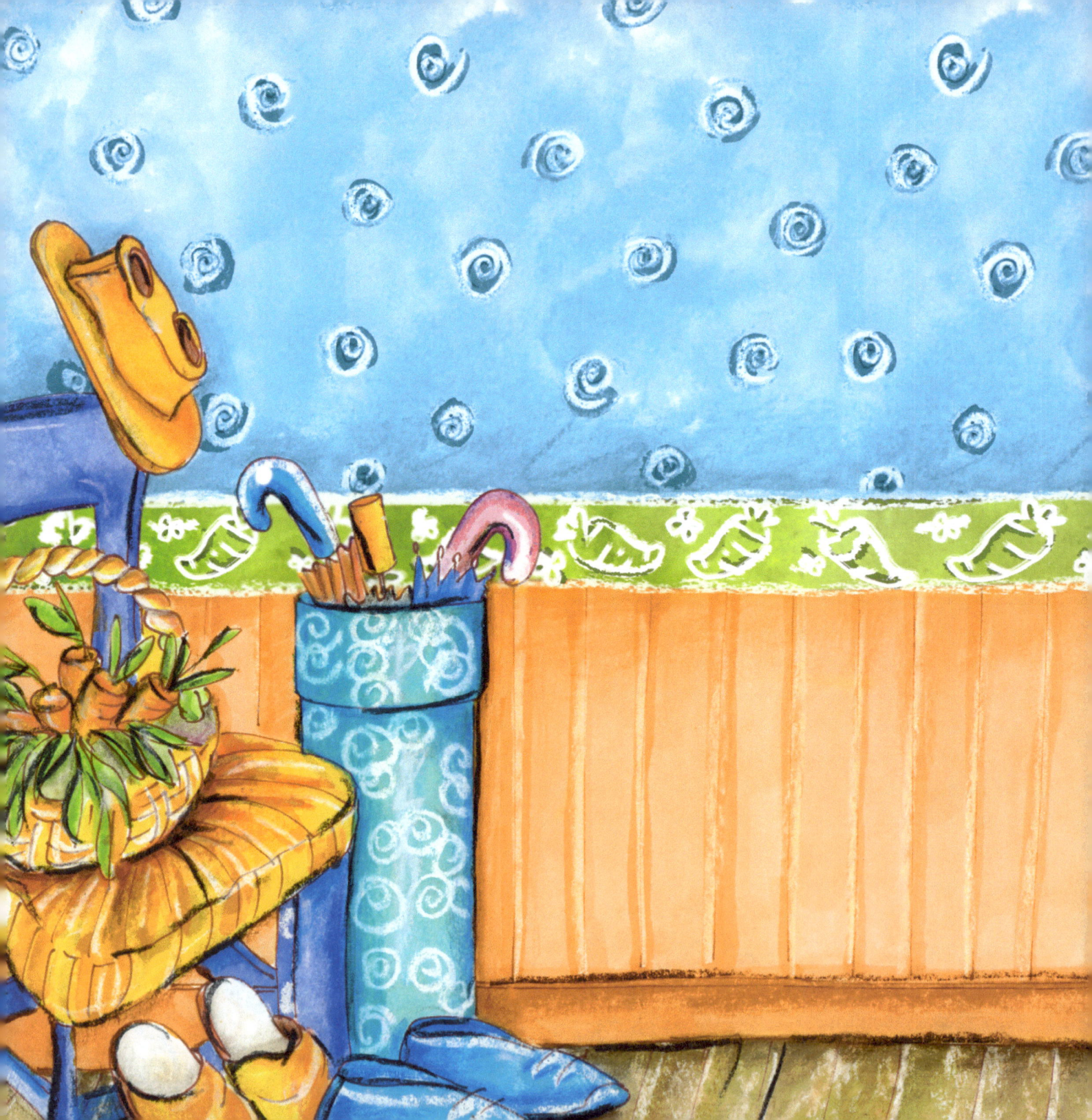

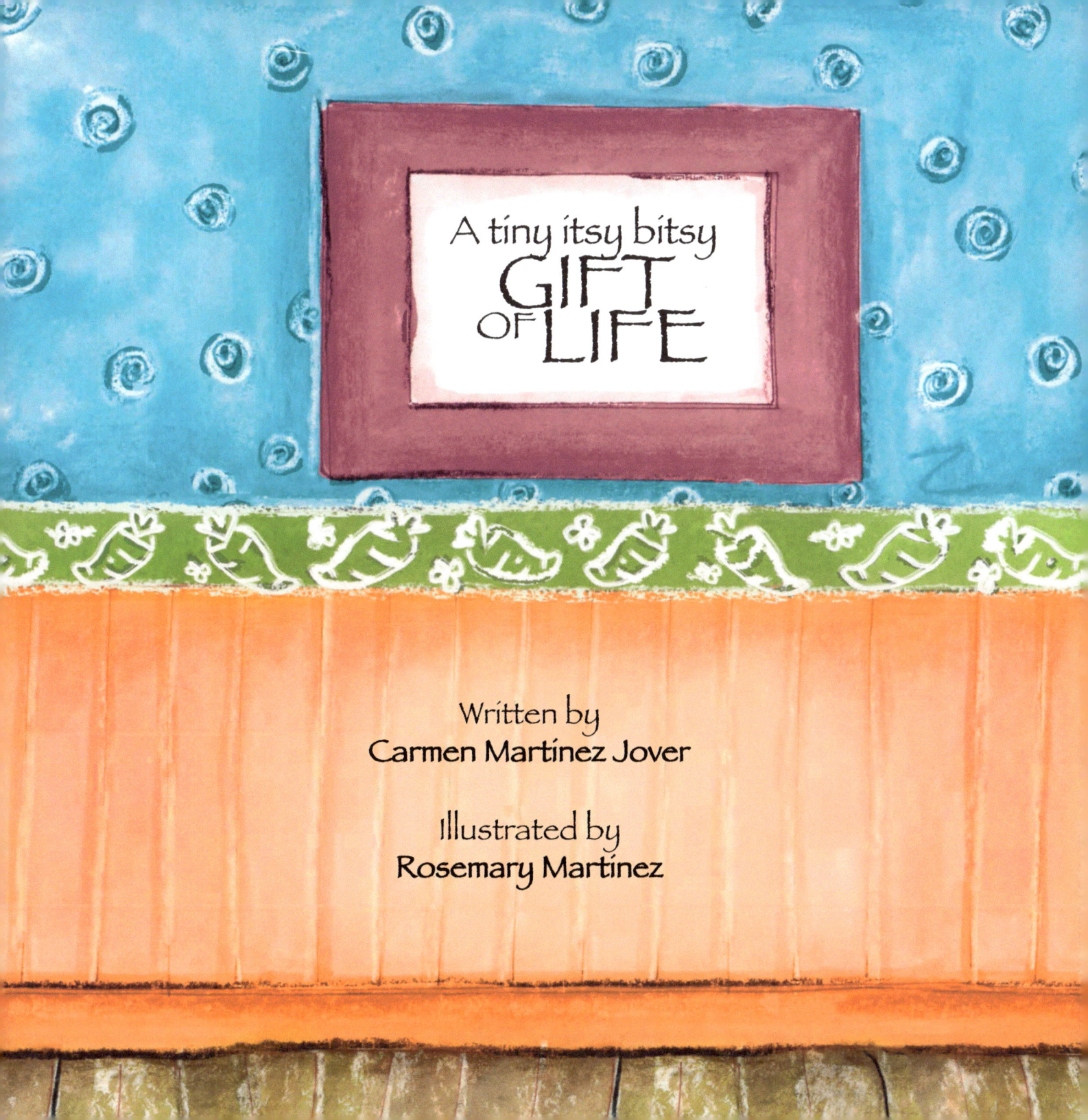

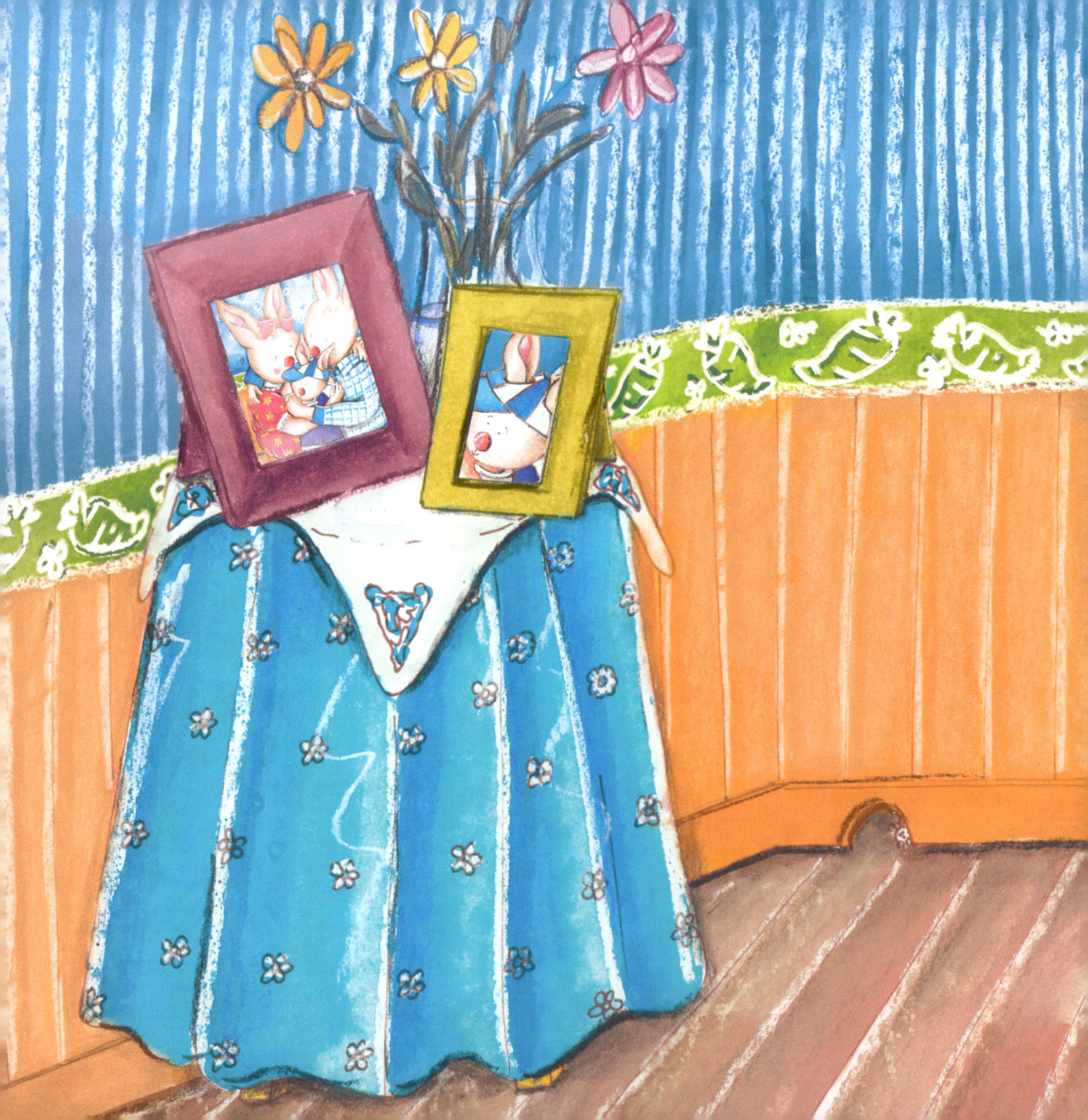

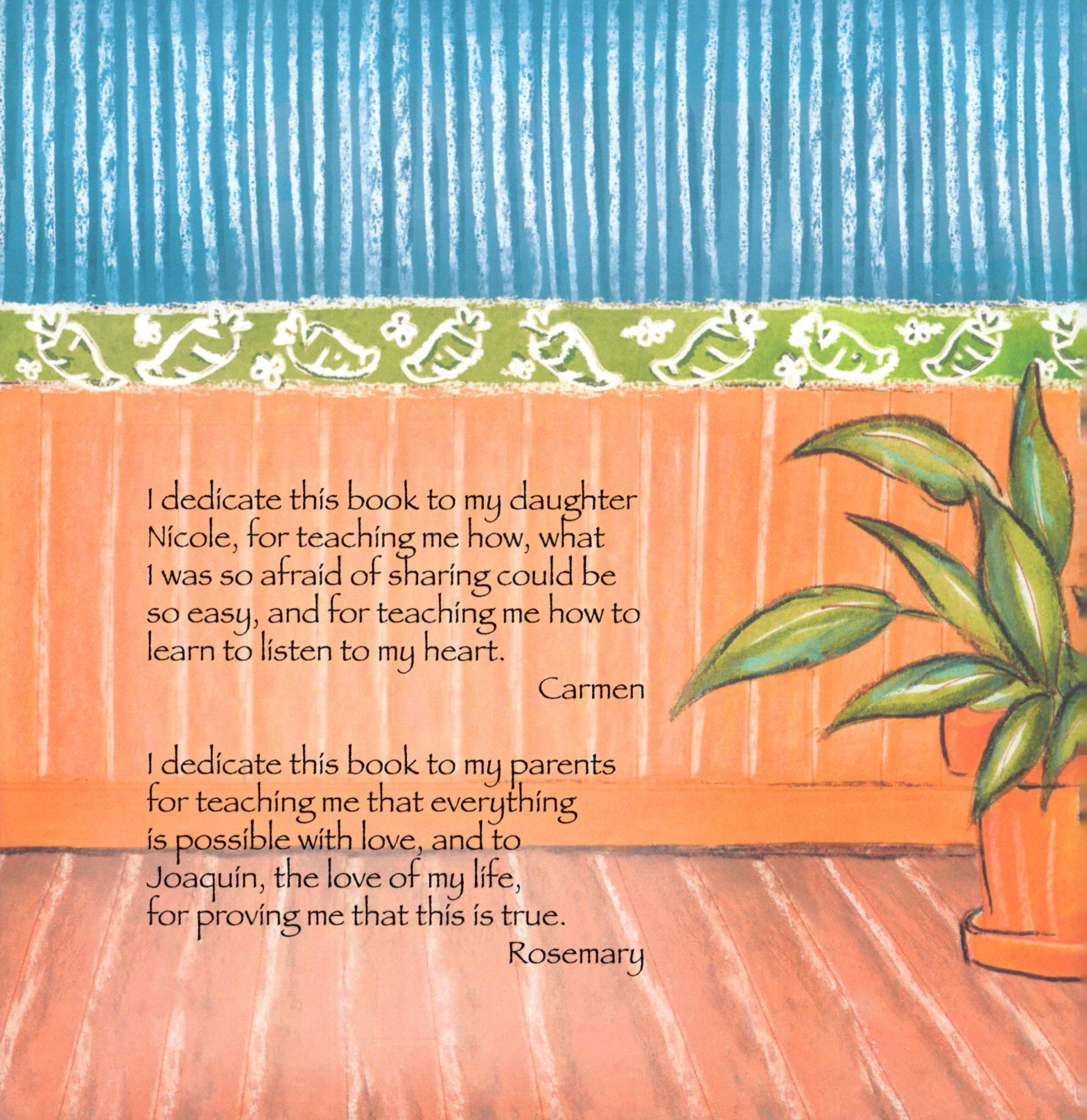

I dedicate this book to my daughter Nicole, for teaching me how, what I was so afraid of sharing could be so easy, and for teaching me how to learn to listen to my heart.

                                     Carmen

I dedicate this book to my parents for teaching me that everything is possible with love, and to Joaquin, the love of my life, for proving me that this is true.

                                     Rosemary

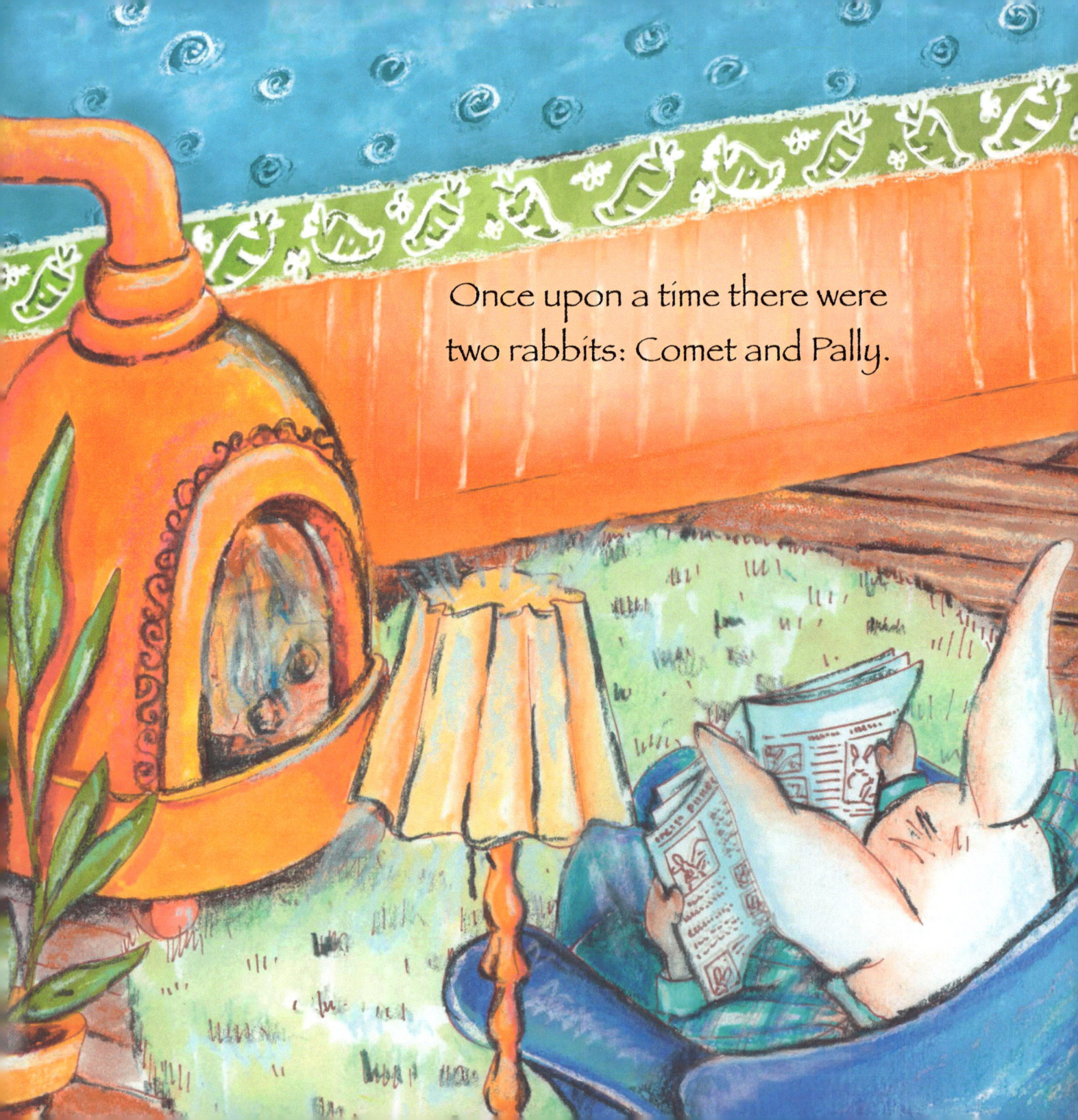

Once upon a time there were two rabbits: Comet and Pally.

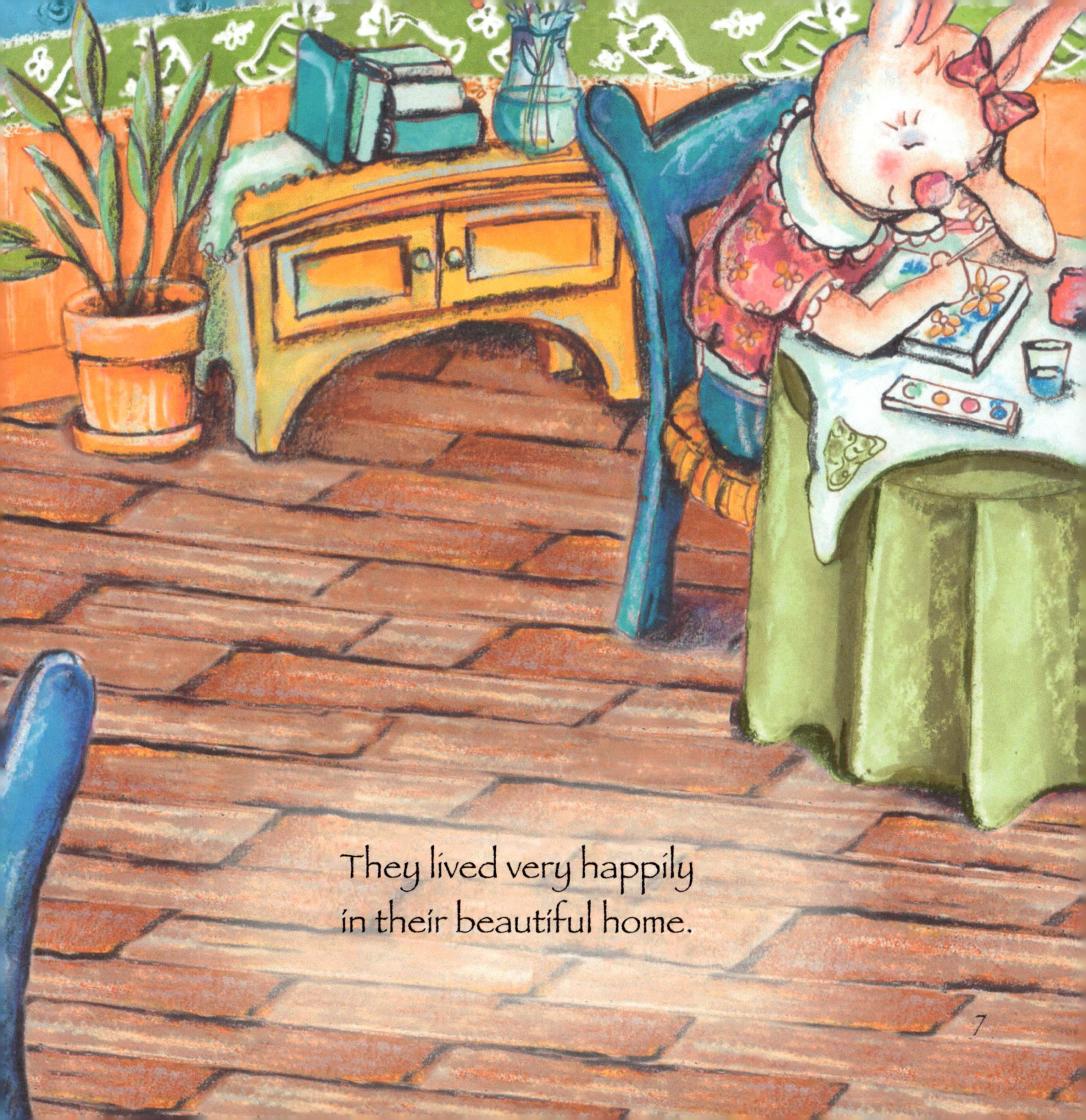

They lived very happily
in their beautiful home.

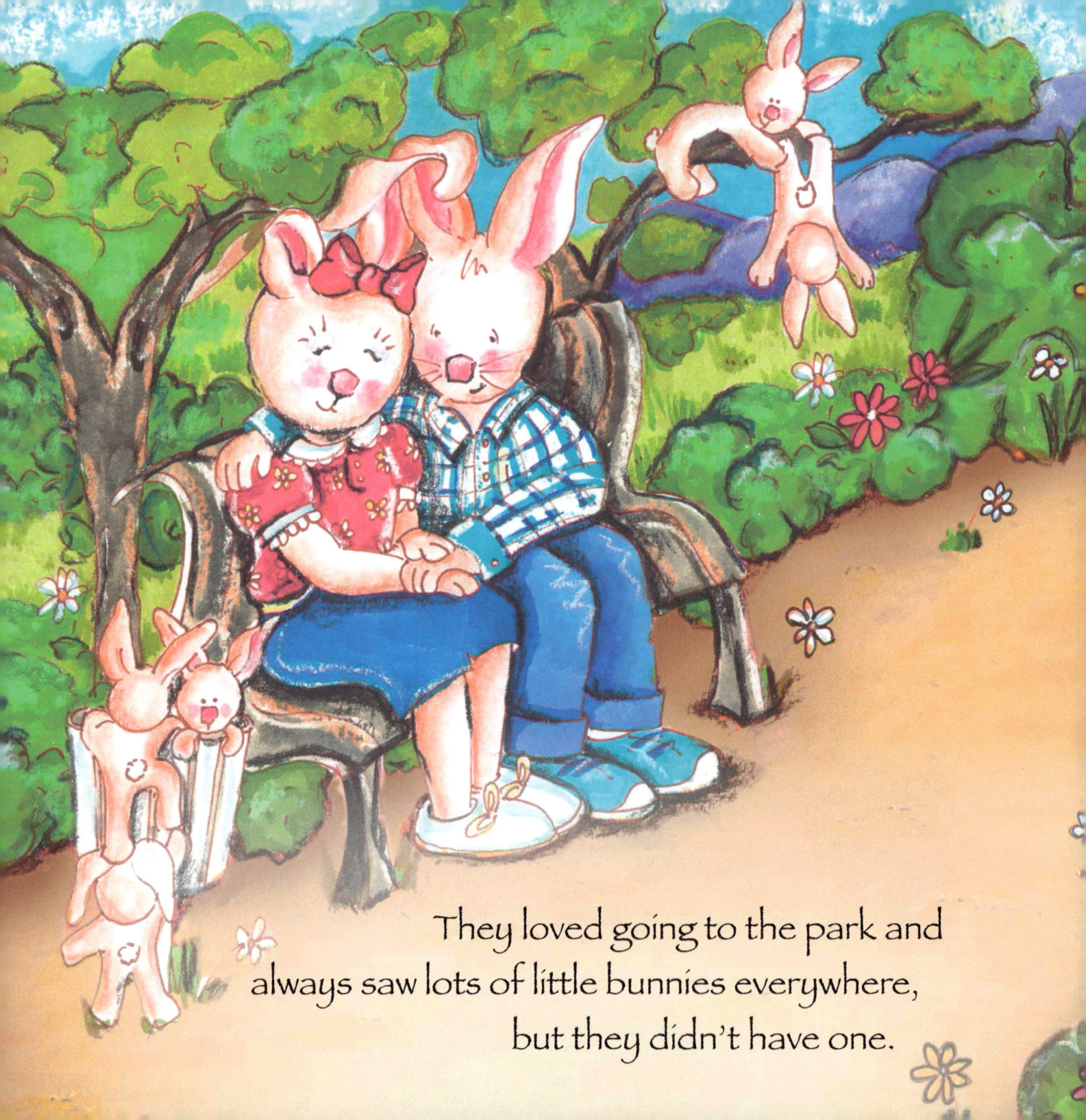

They loved going to the park and always saw lots of little bunnies everywhere, but they didn't have one.

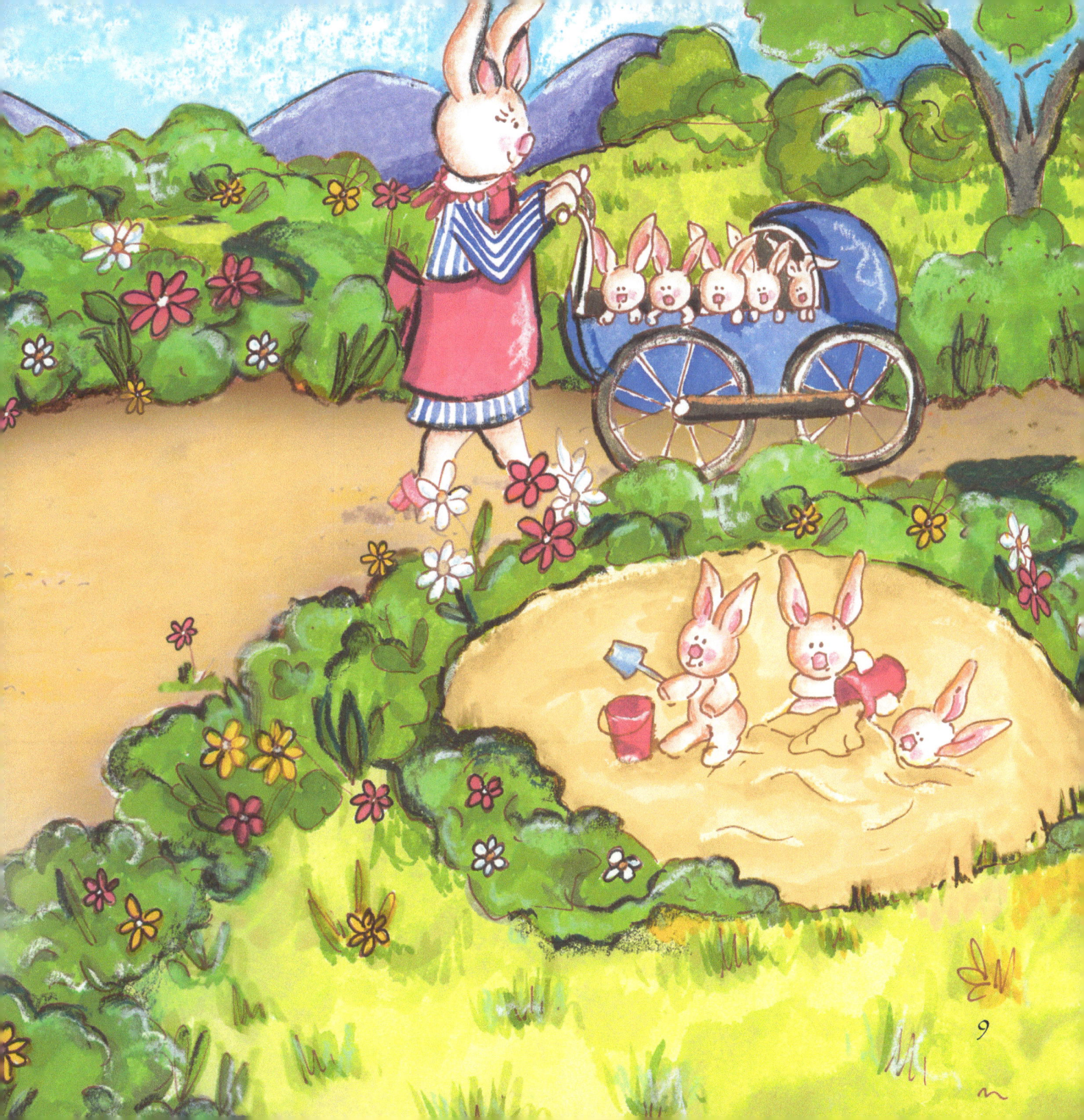

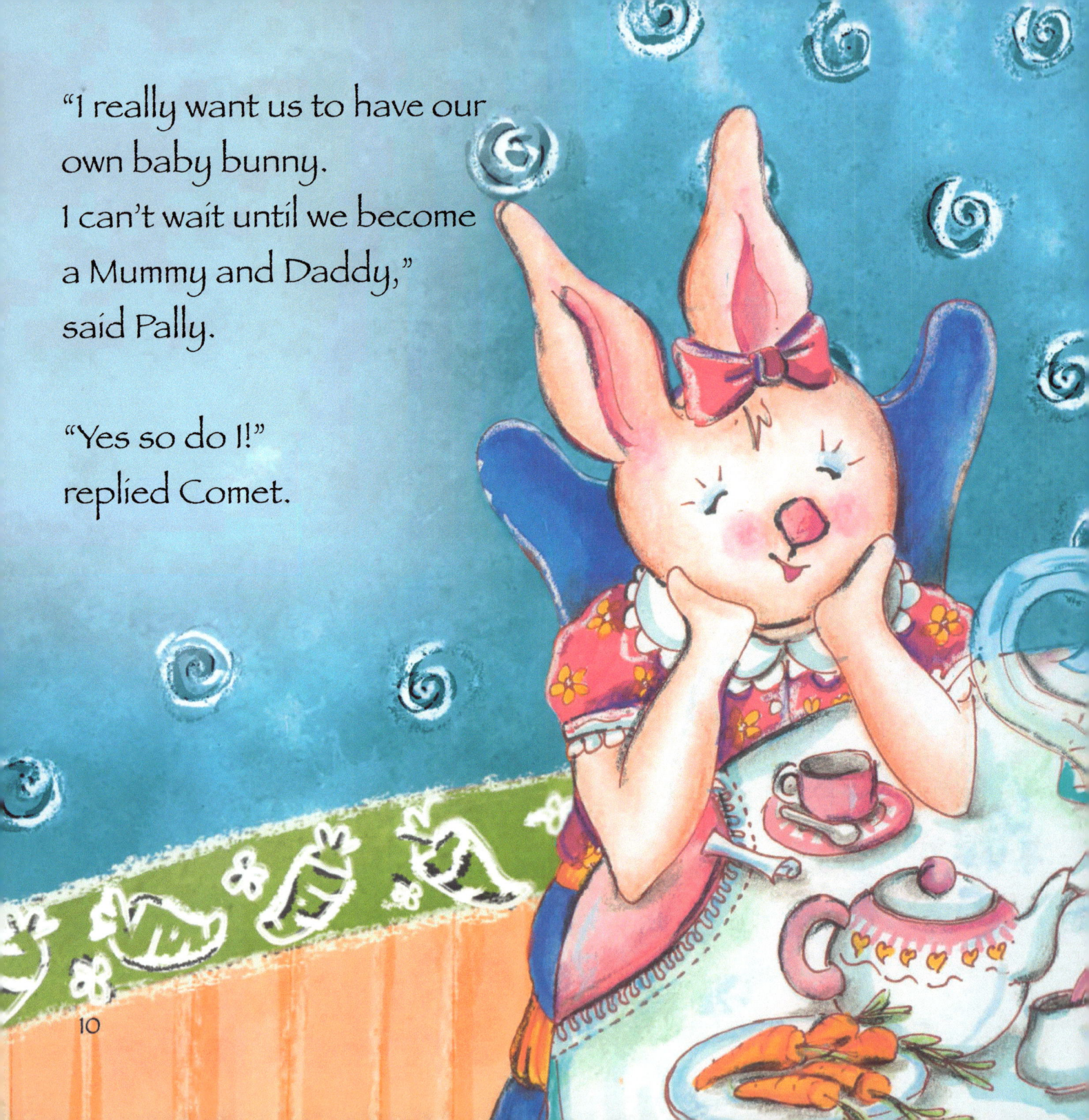

"I really want us to have our own baby bunny. I can't wait until we become a Mummy and Daddy," said Pally.

"Yes so do I!" replied Comet.

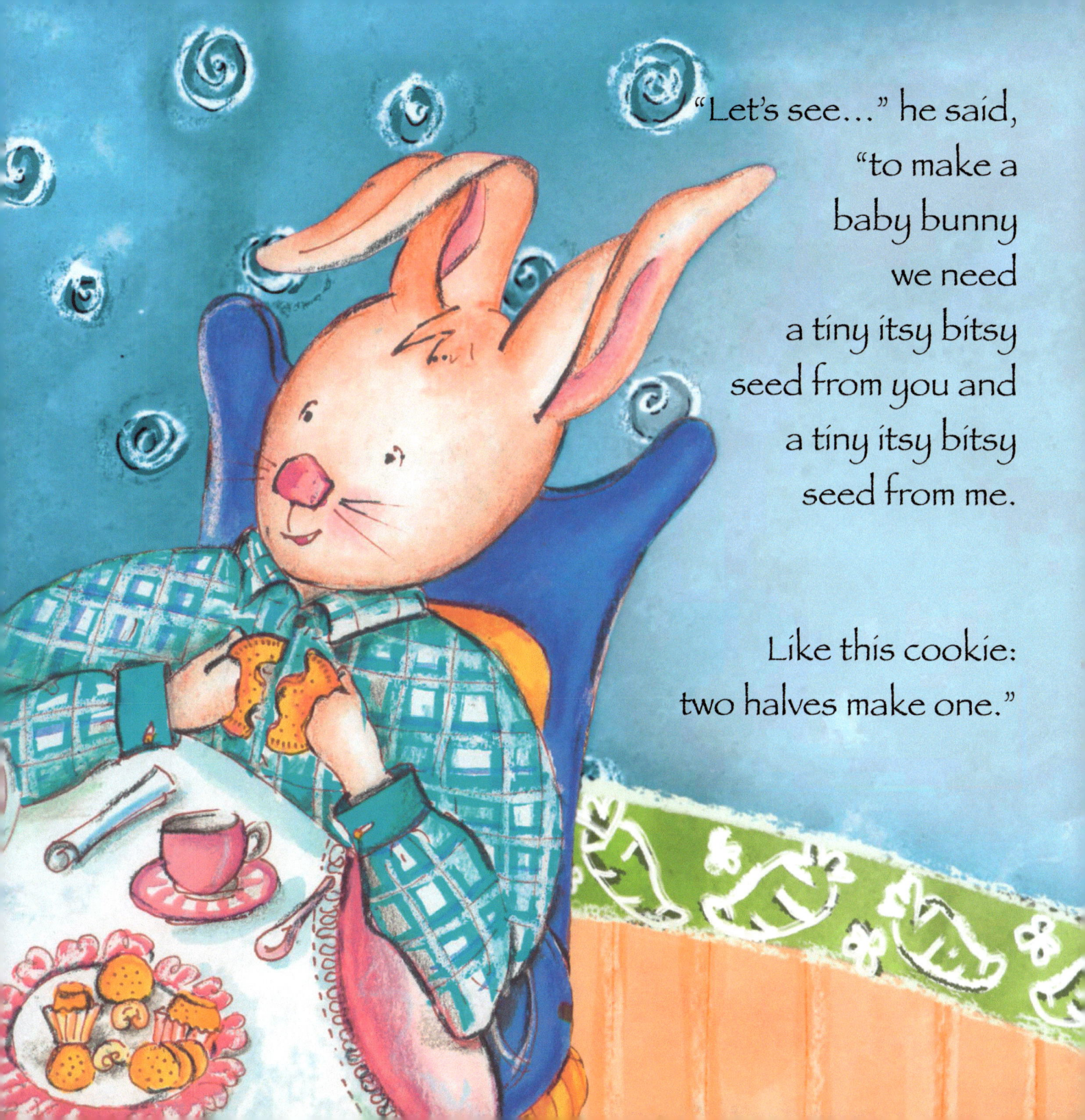

"Let's see…" he said, "to make a baby bunny we need a tiny itsy bitsy seed from you and a tiny itsy bitsy seed from me.

Like this cookie: two halves make one."

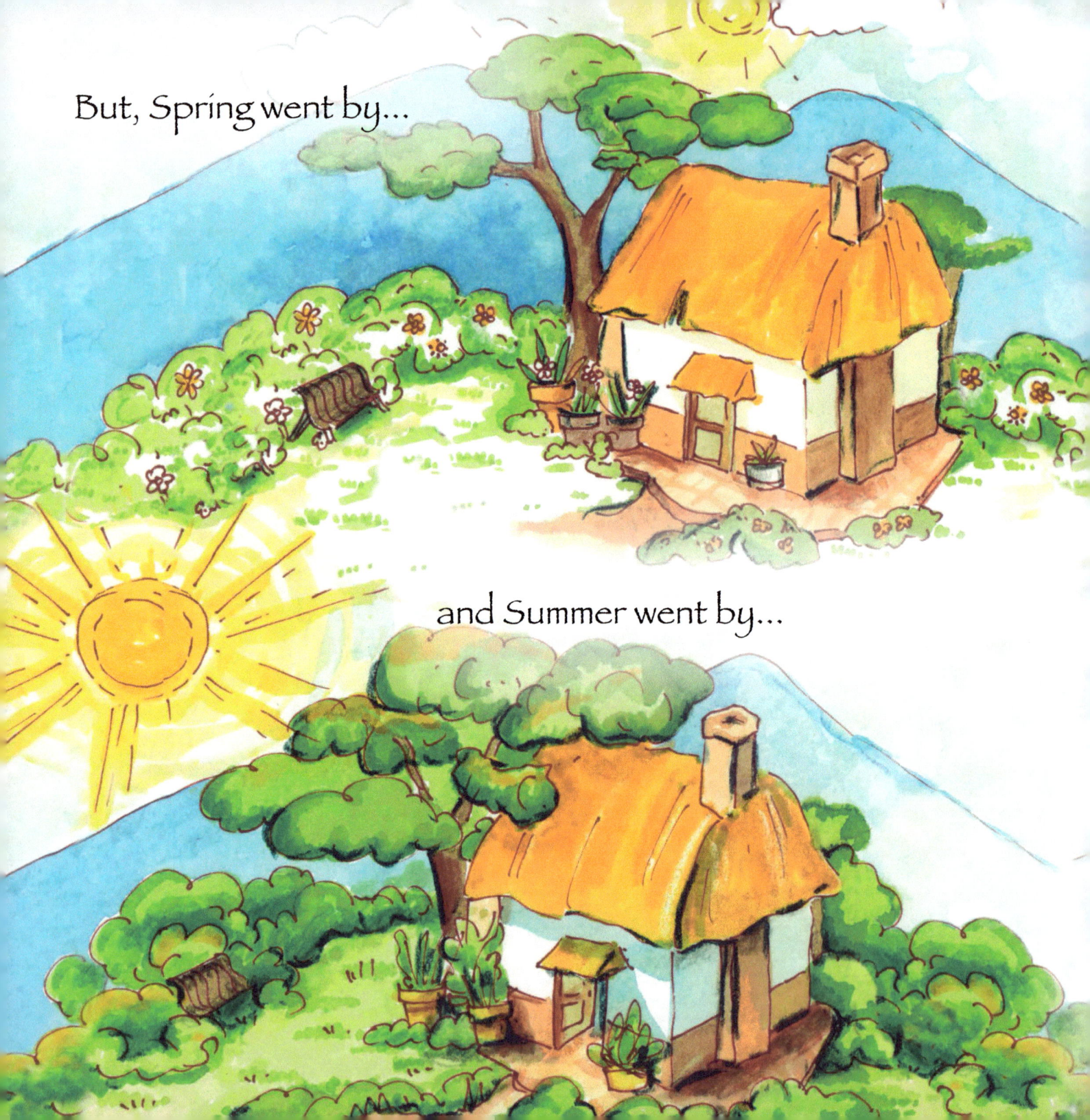

But, Spring went by...

and Summer went by...

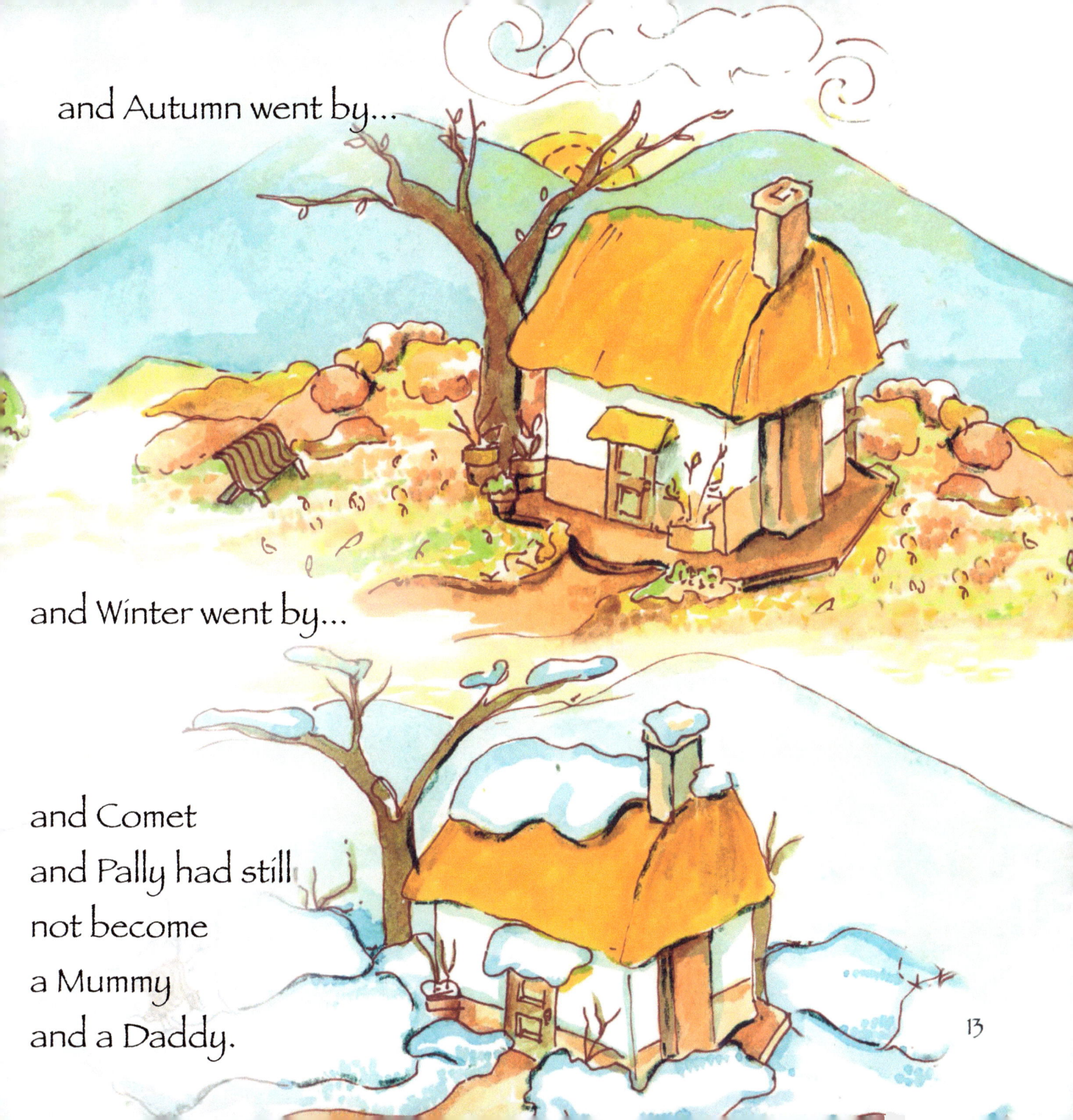

and Autumn went by...

and Winter went by...

and Comet and Pally had still not become a Mummy and a Daddy.

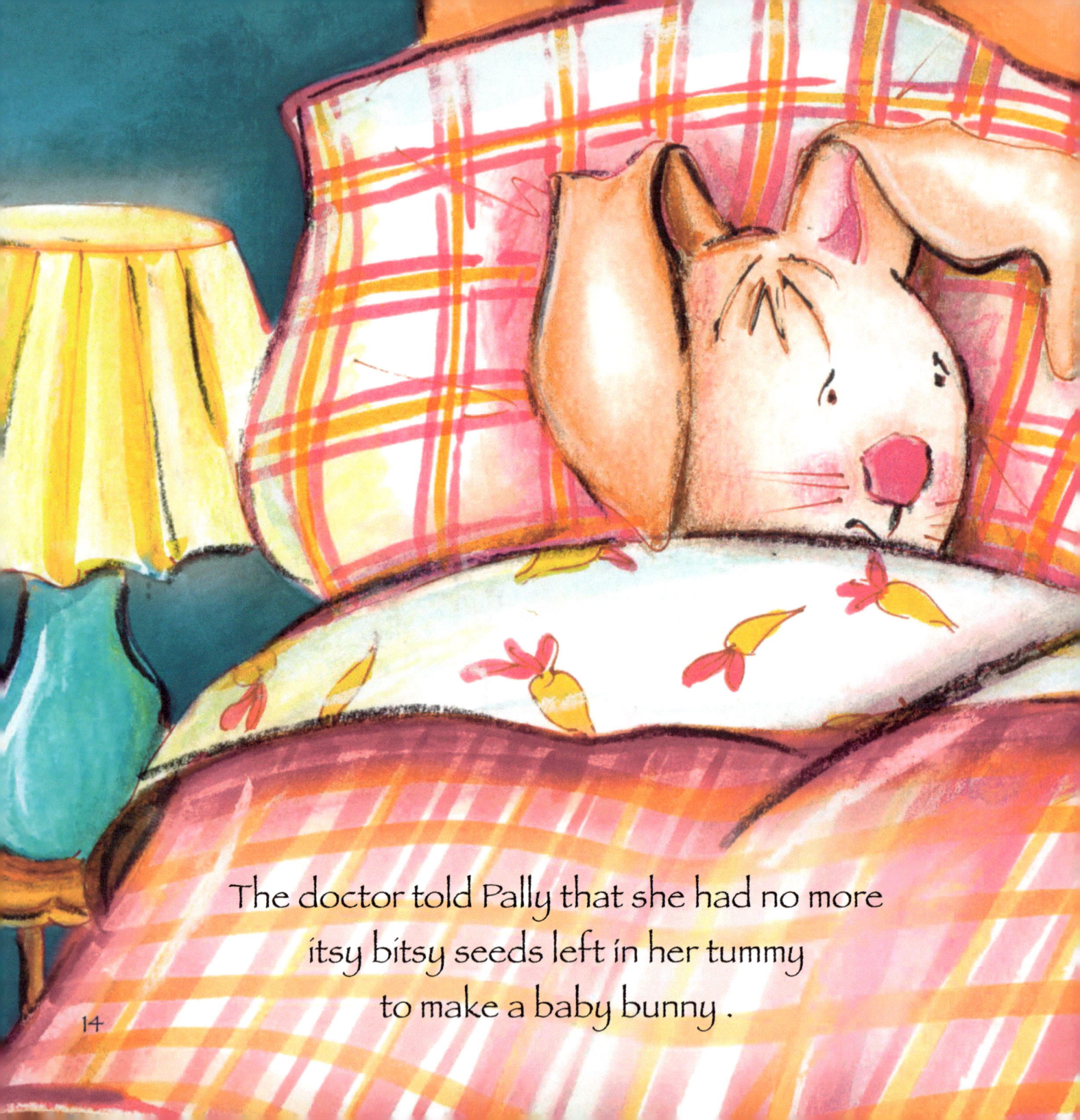

The doctor told Pally that she had no more itsy bitsy seeds left in her tummy to make a baby bunny.

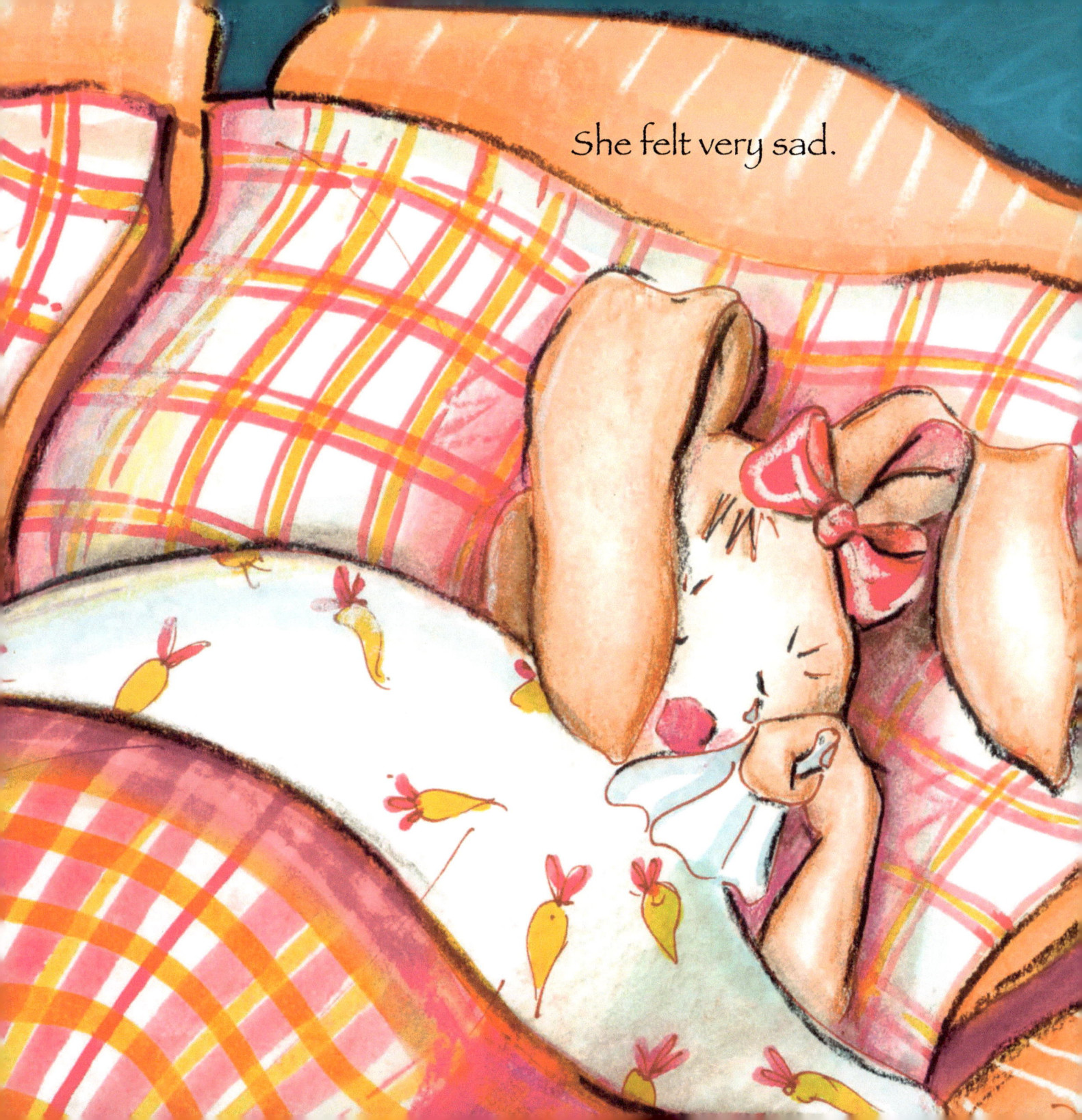
She felt very sad.

One special sunny day, a lady rabbit knocked on the door.

They had never seen her before.

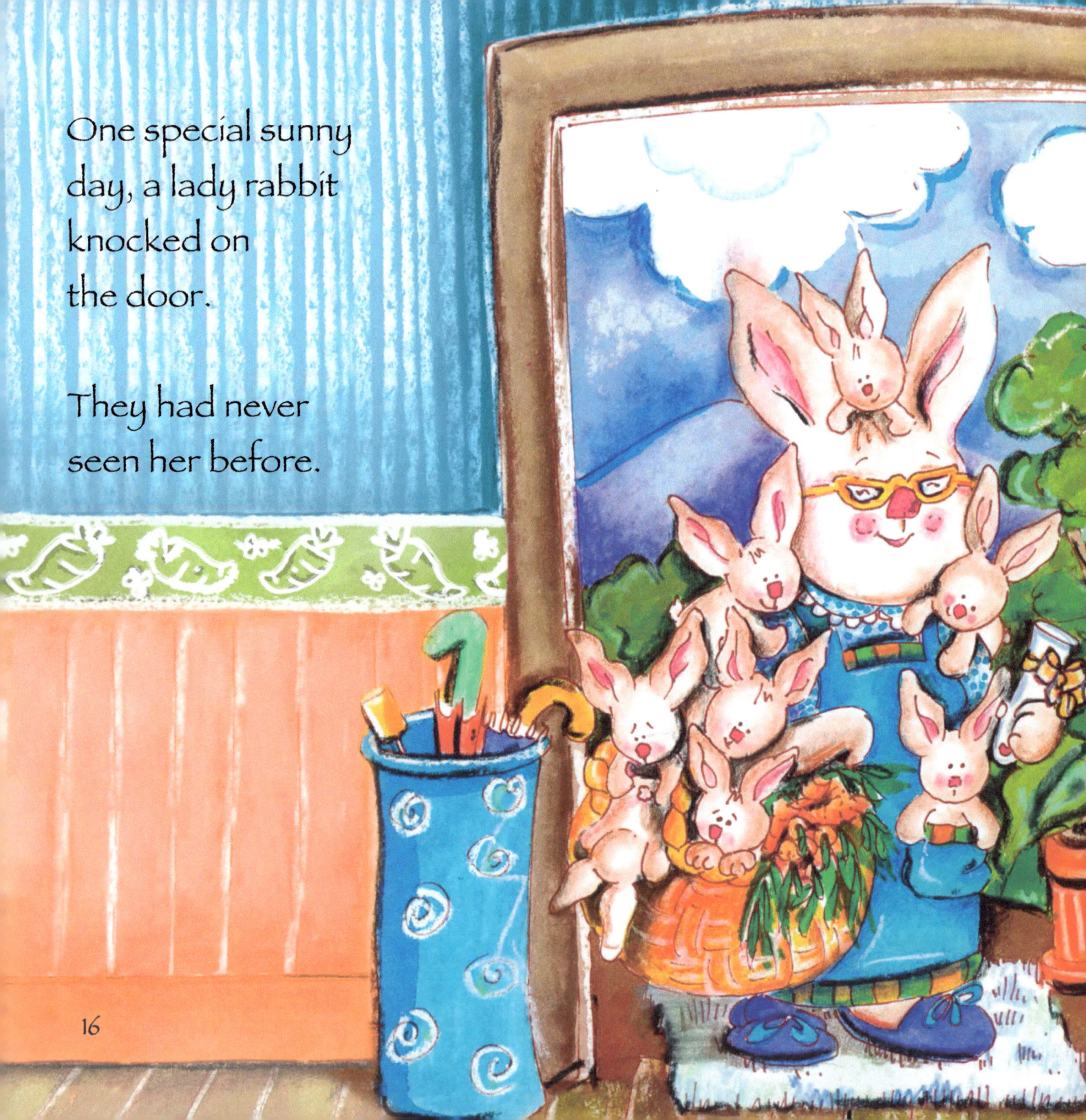

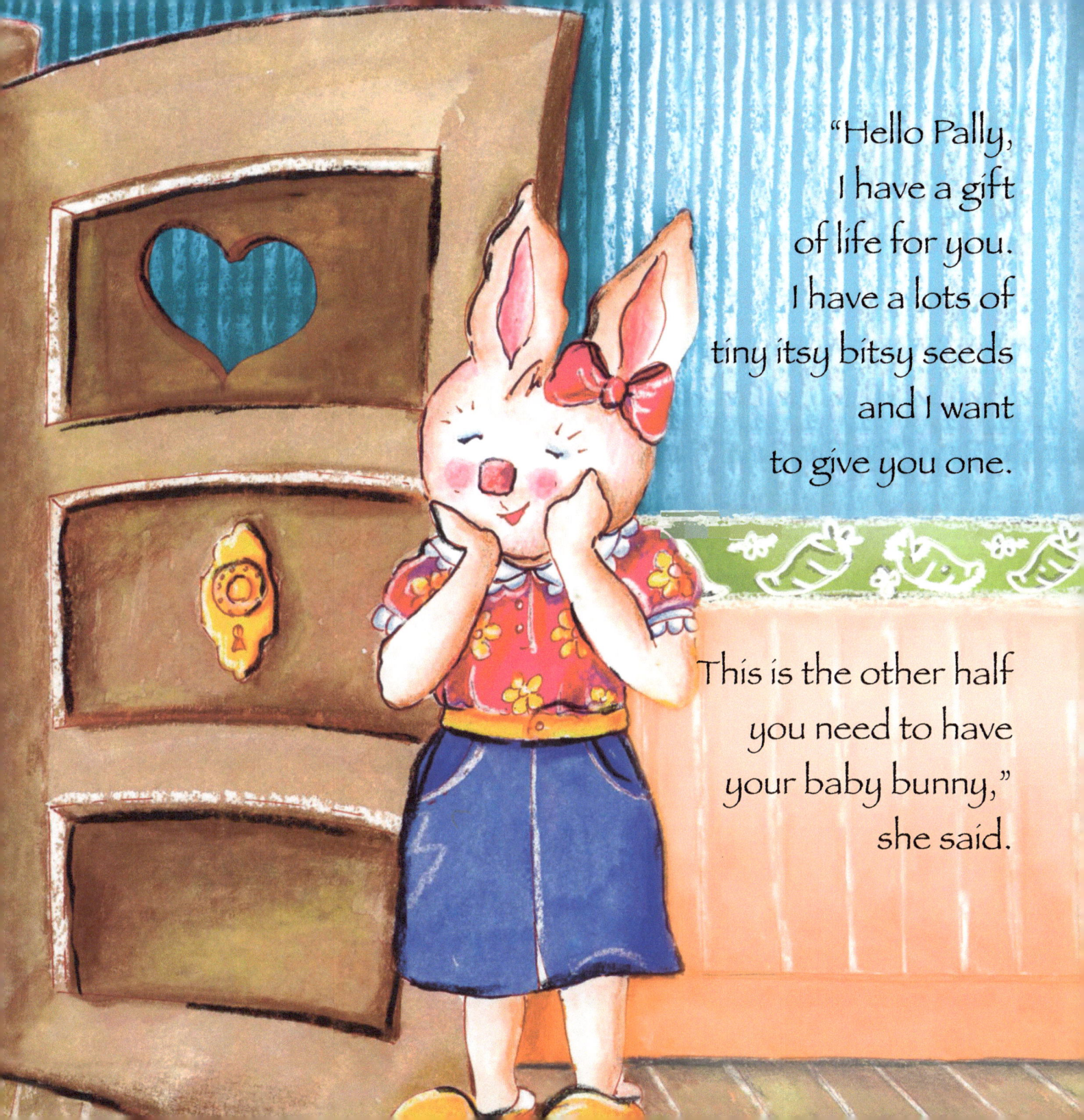

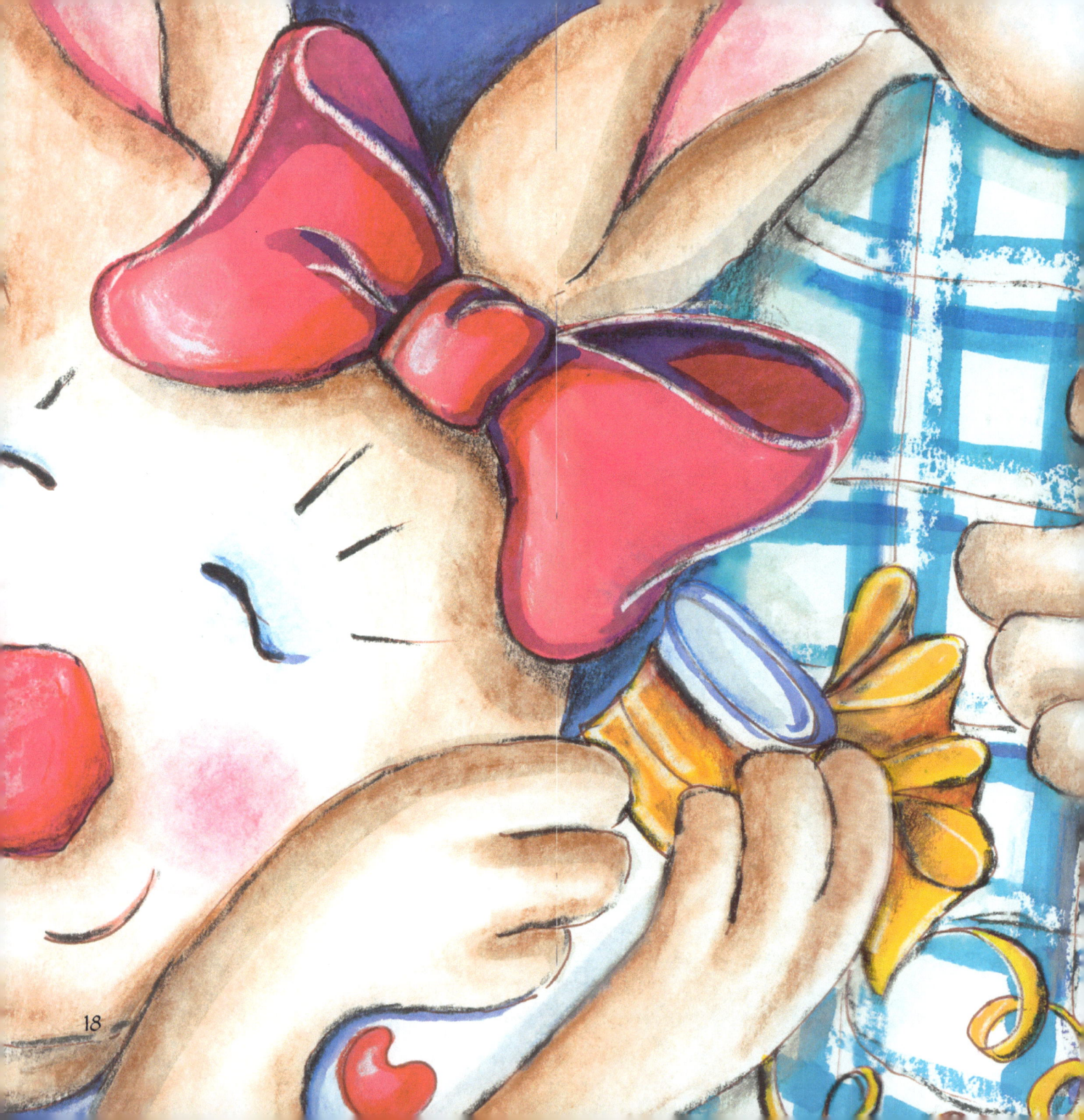

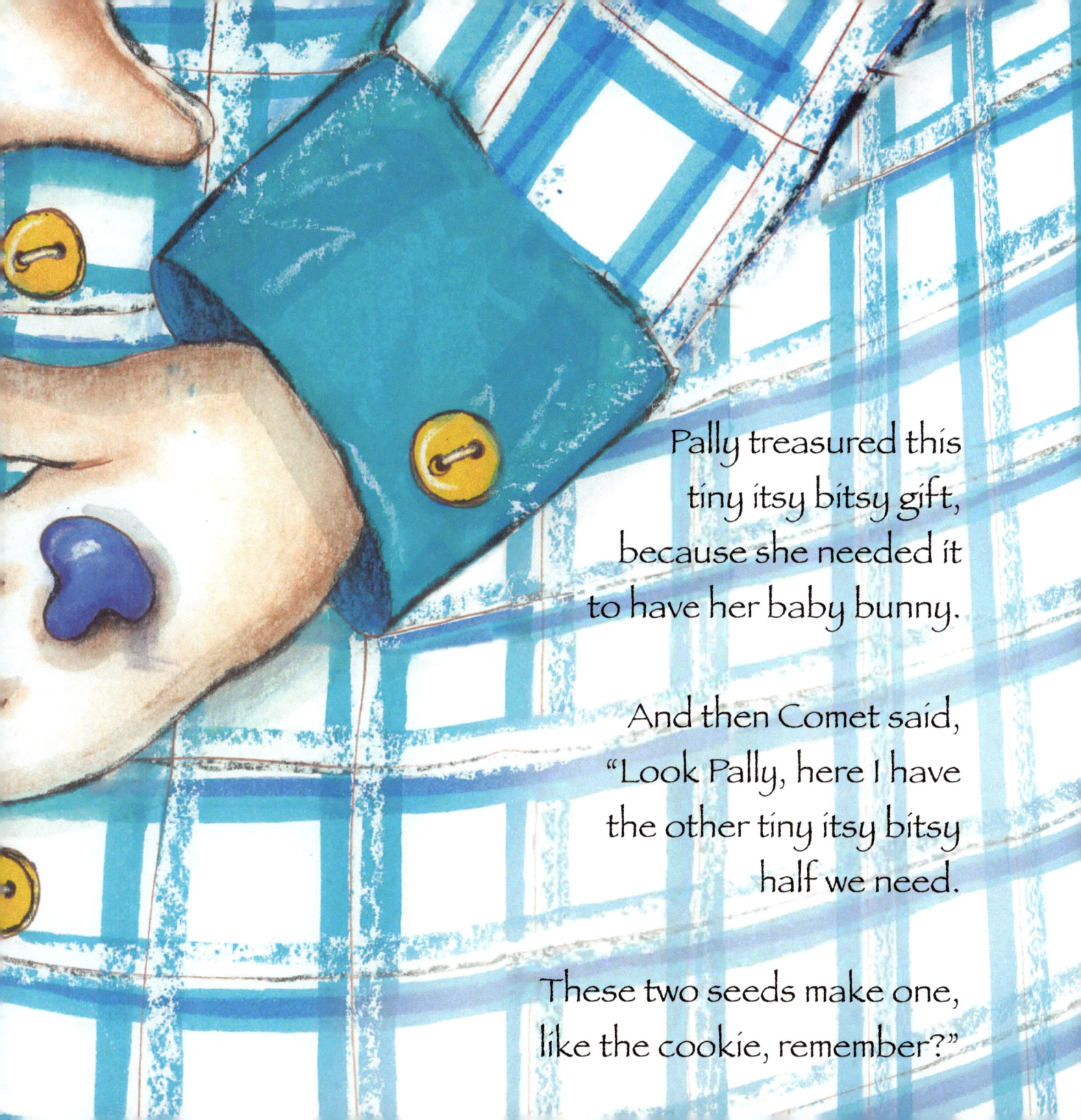

Pally treasured this tiny itsy bitsy gift, because she needed it to have her baby bunny.

And then Comet said, "Look Pally, here I have the other tiny itsy bitsy half we need.

These two seeds make one, like the cookie, remember?"

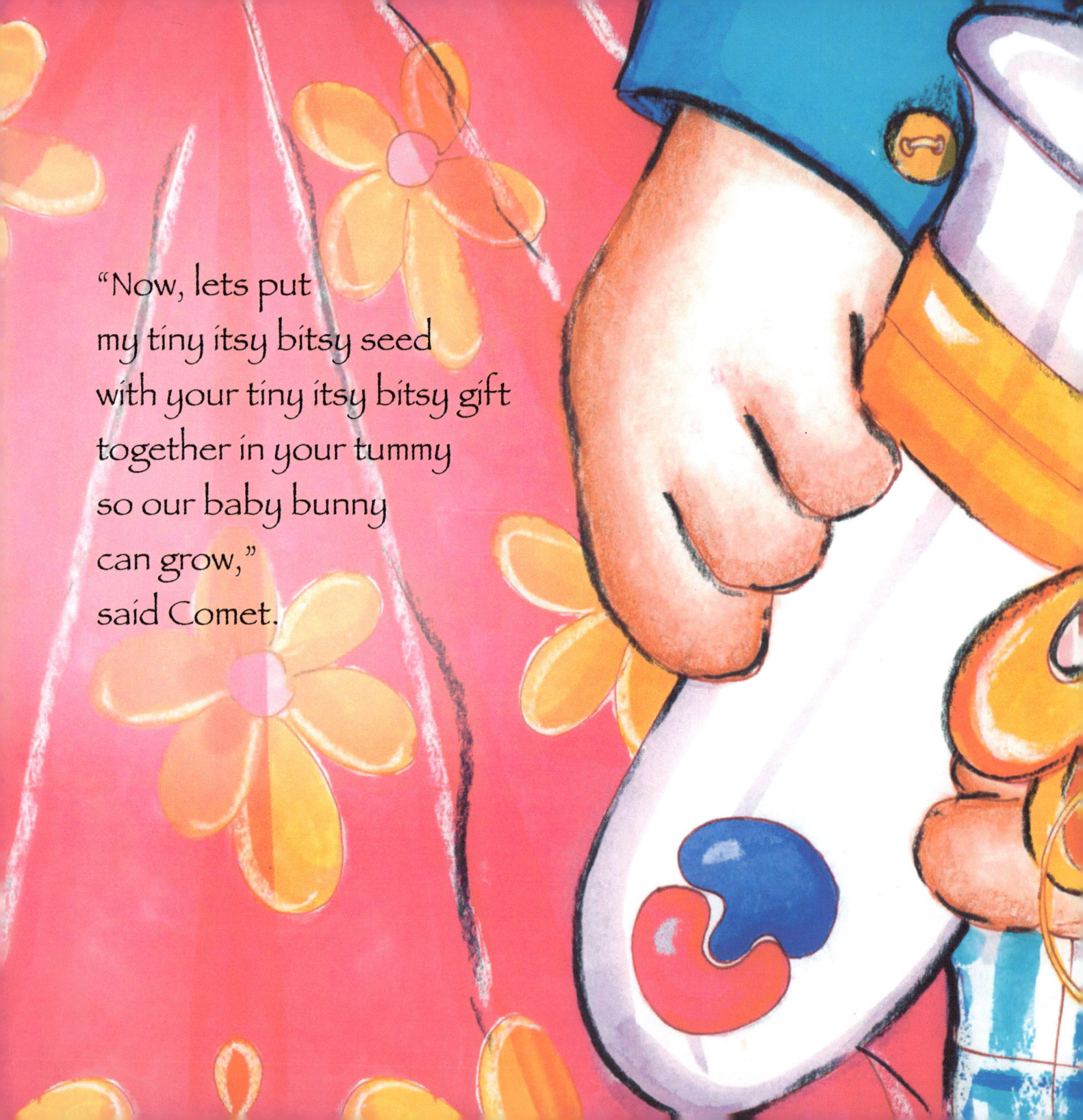

"Now, lets put
my tiny itsy bitsy seed
with your tiny itsy bitsy gift
together in your tummy
so our baby bunny
can grow,"
said Comet.

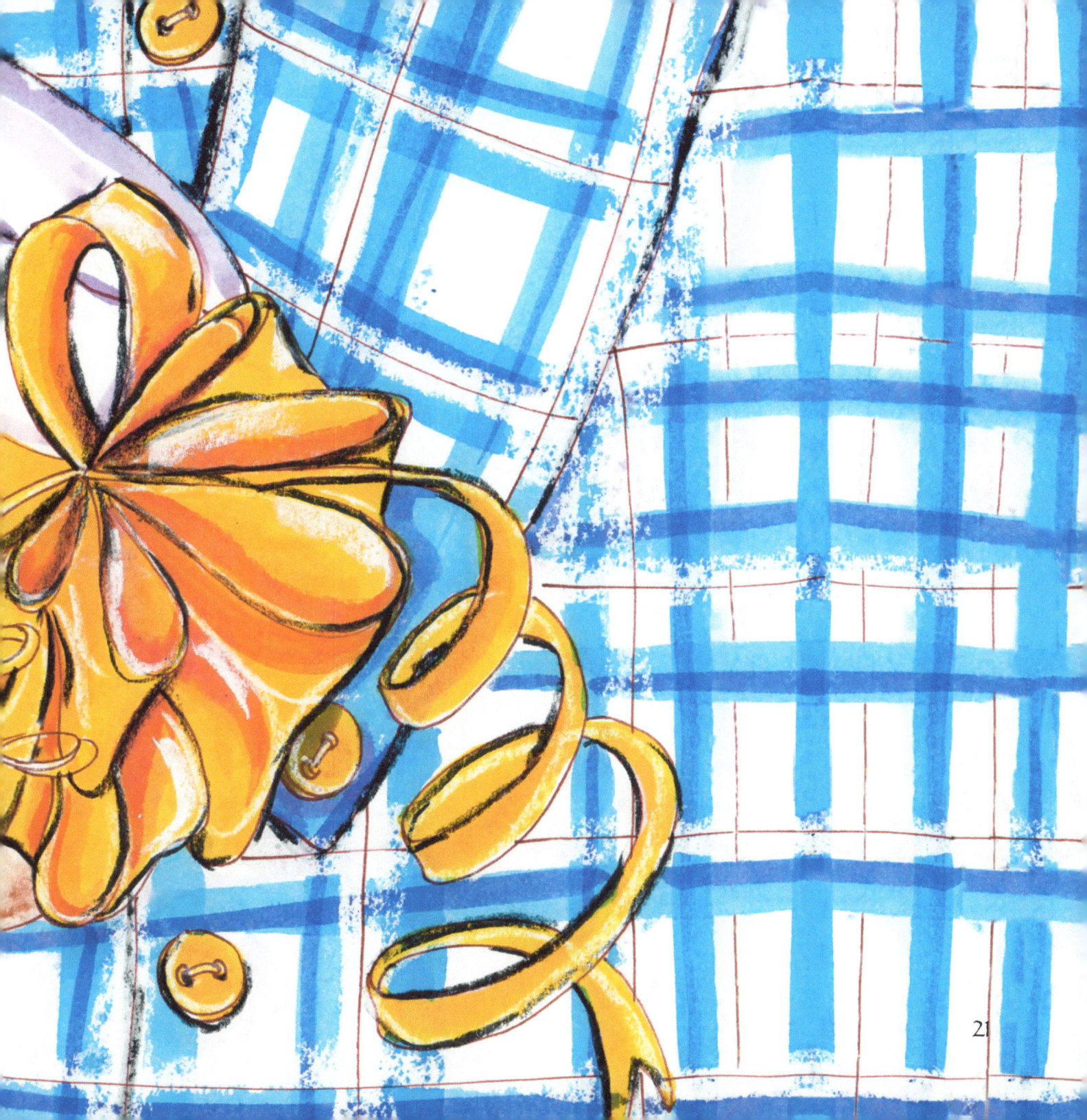

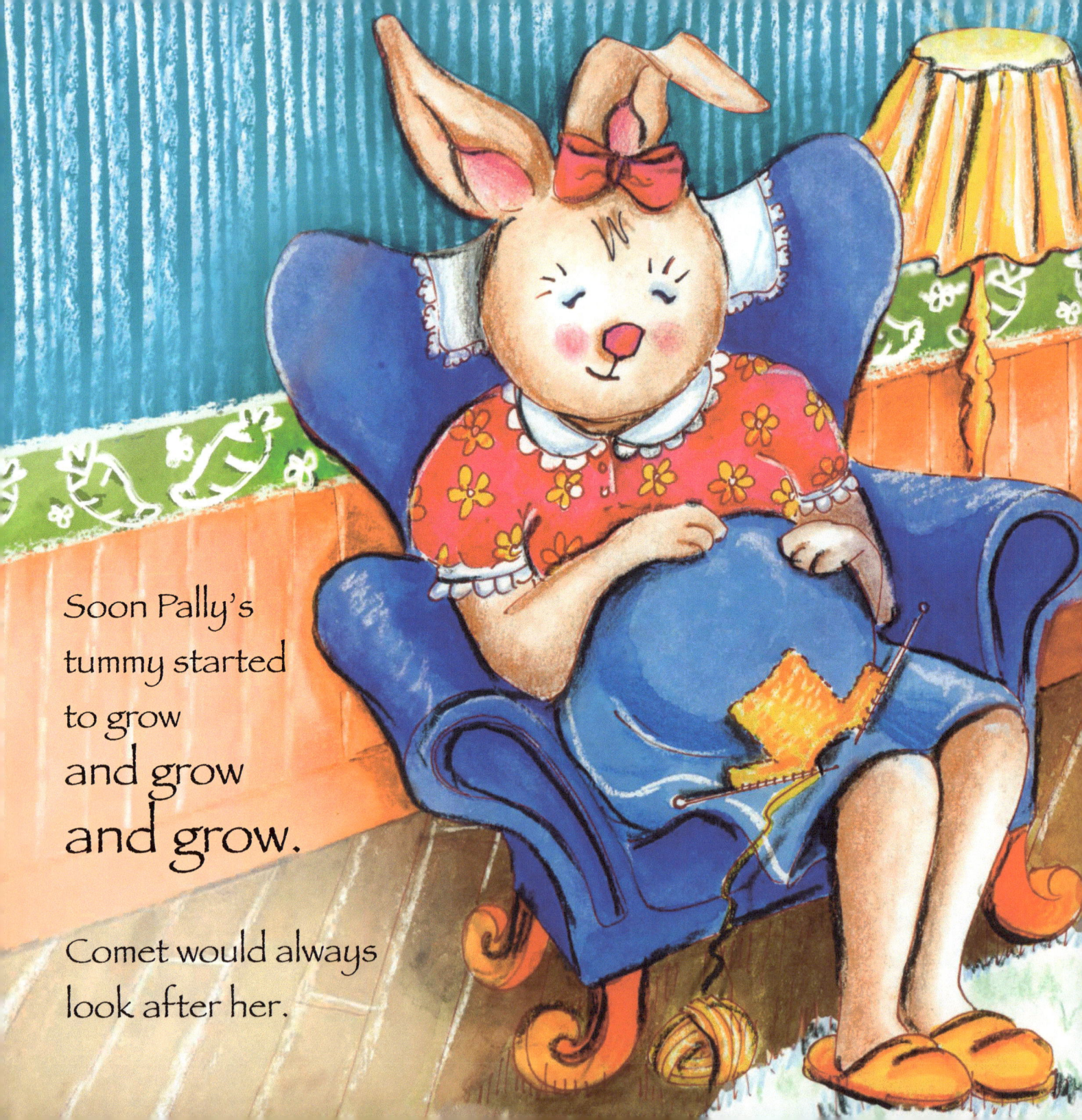

Soon Pally's tummy started to grow and grow and grow.

Comet would always look after her.

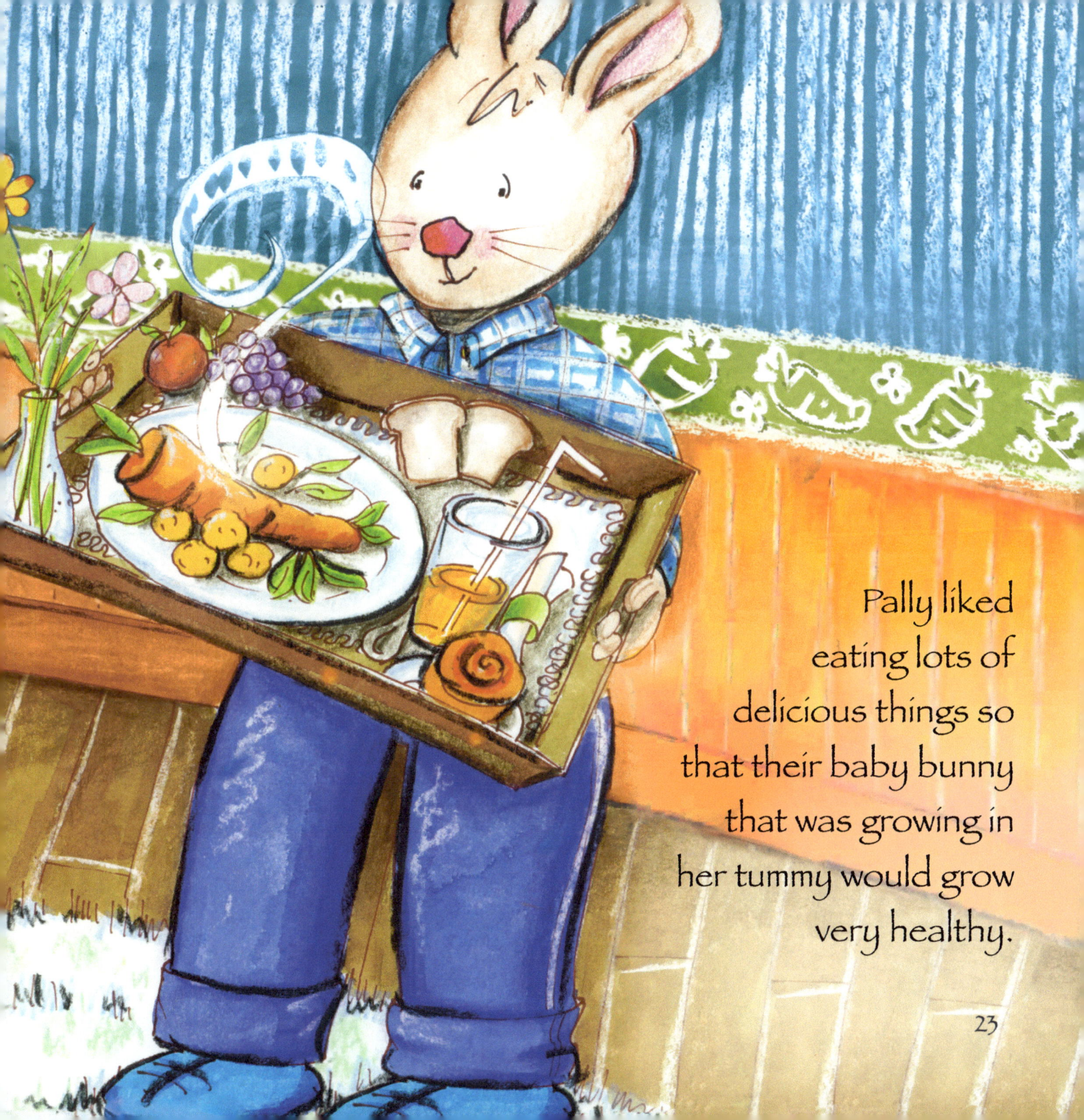

Pally liked eating lots of delicious things so that their baby bunny that was growing in her tummy would grow very healthy.

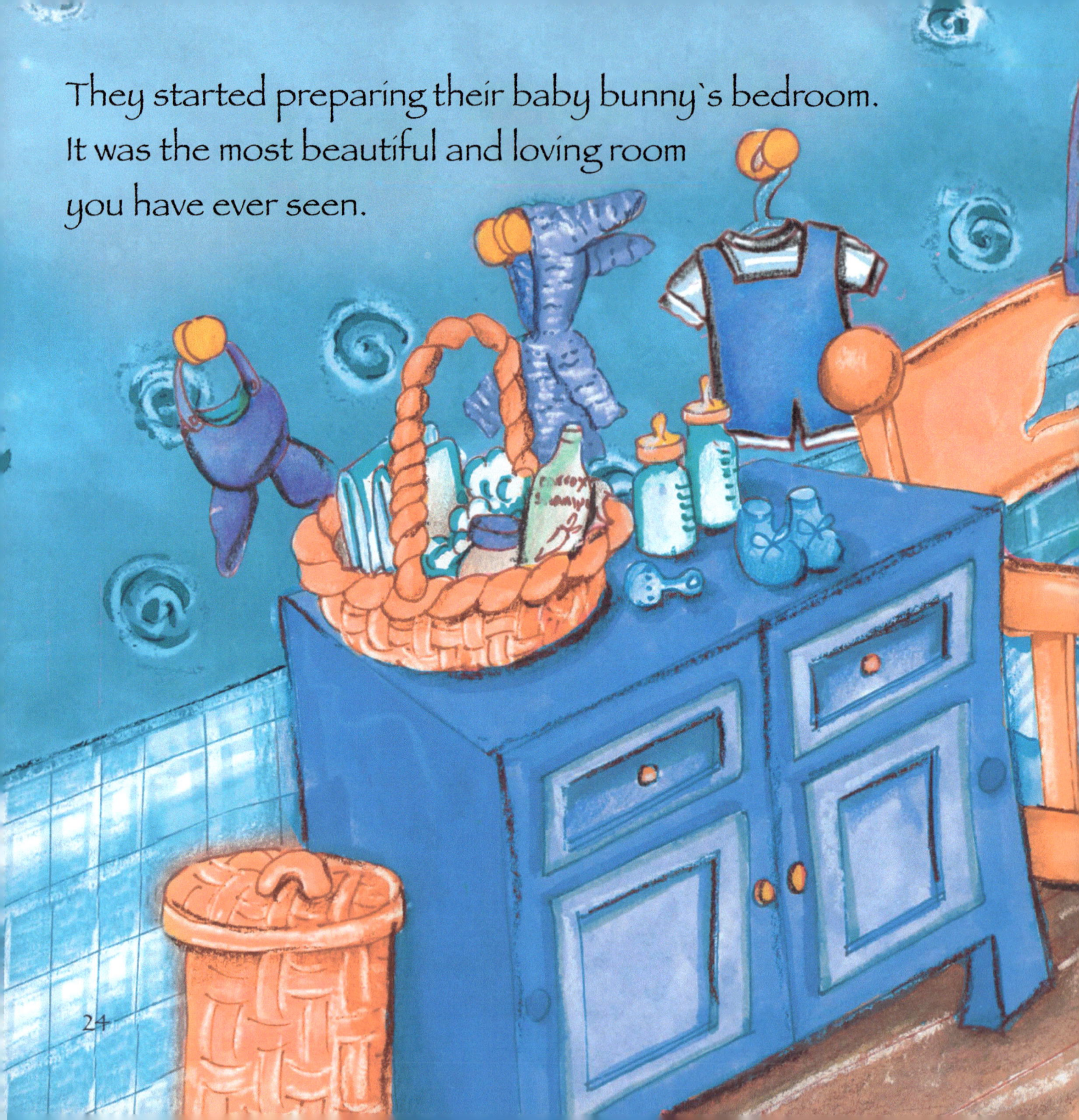

They started preparing their baby bunny's bedroom. It was the most beautiful and loving room you have ever seen.

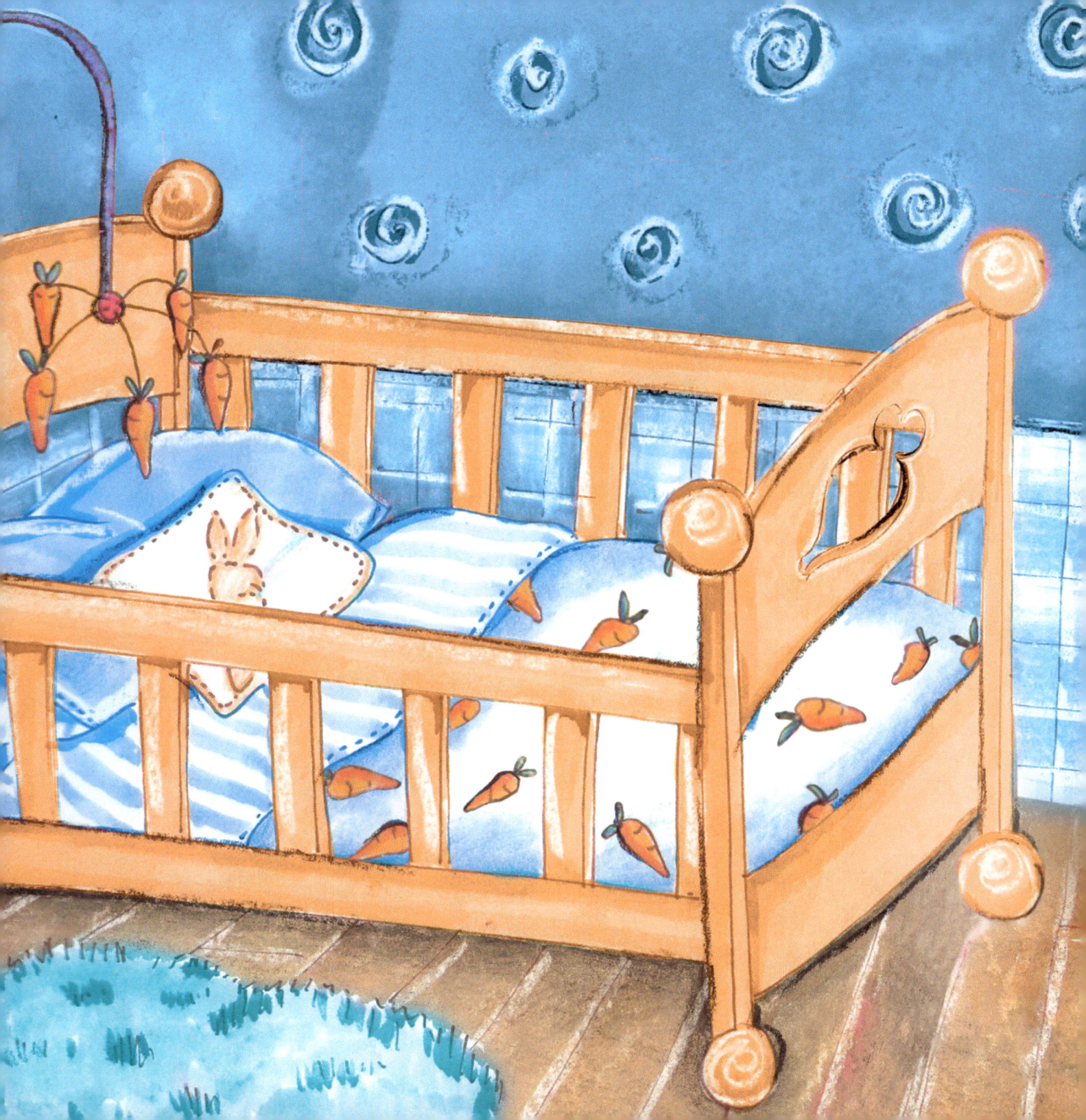

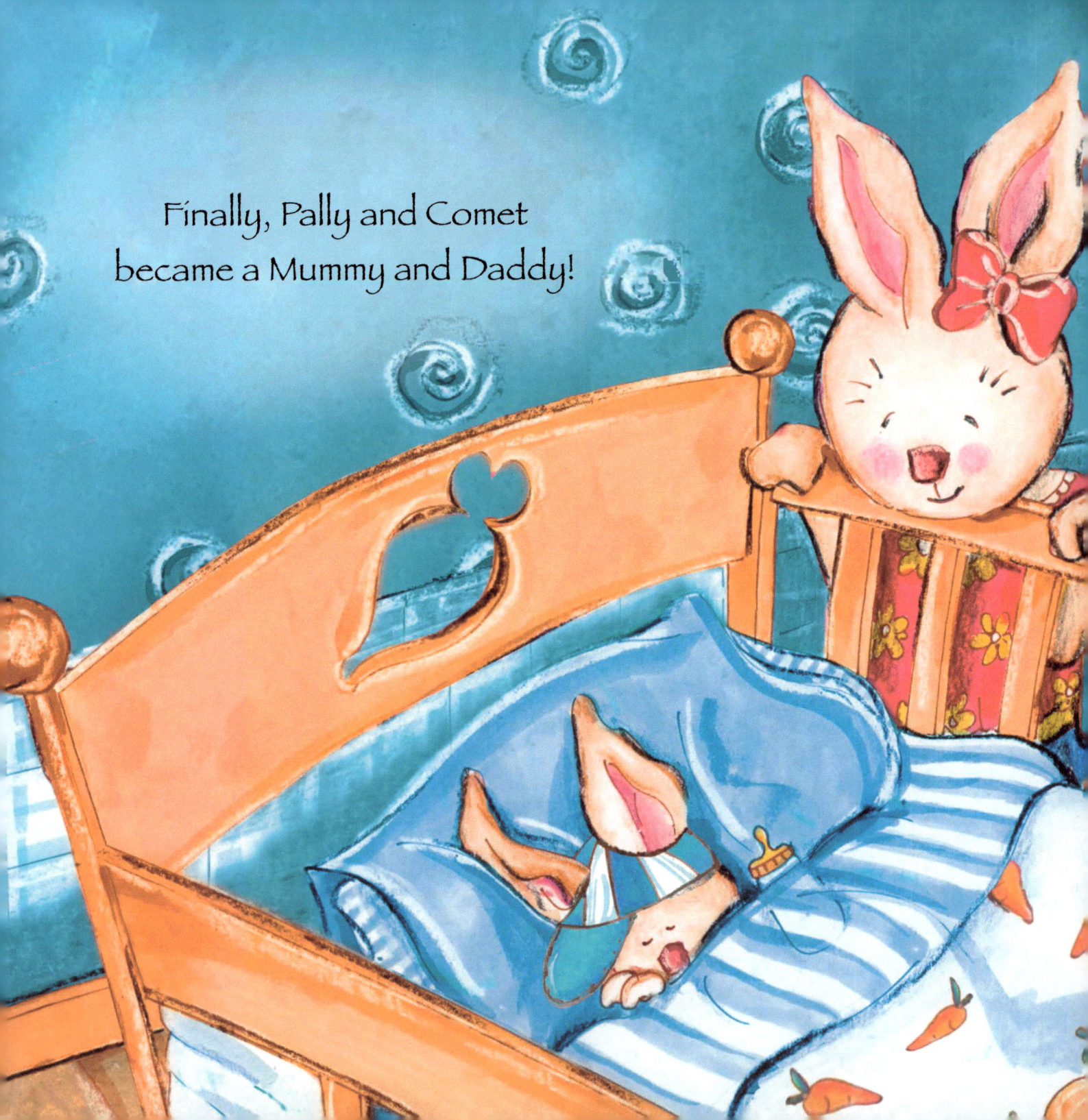
Finally, Pally and Comet became a Mummy and Daddy!

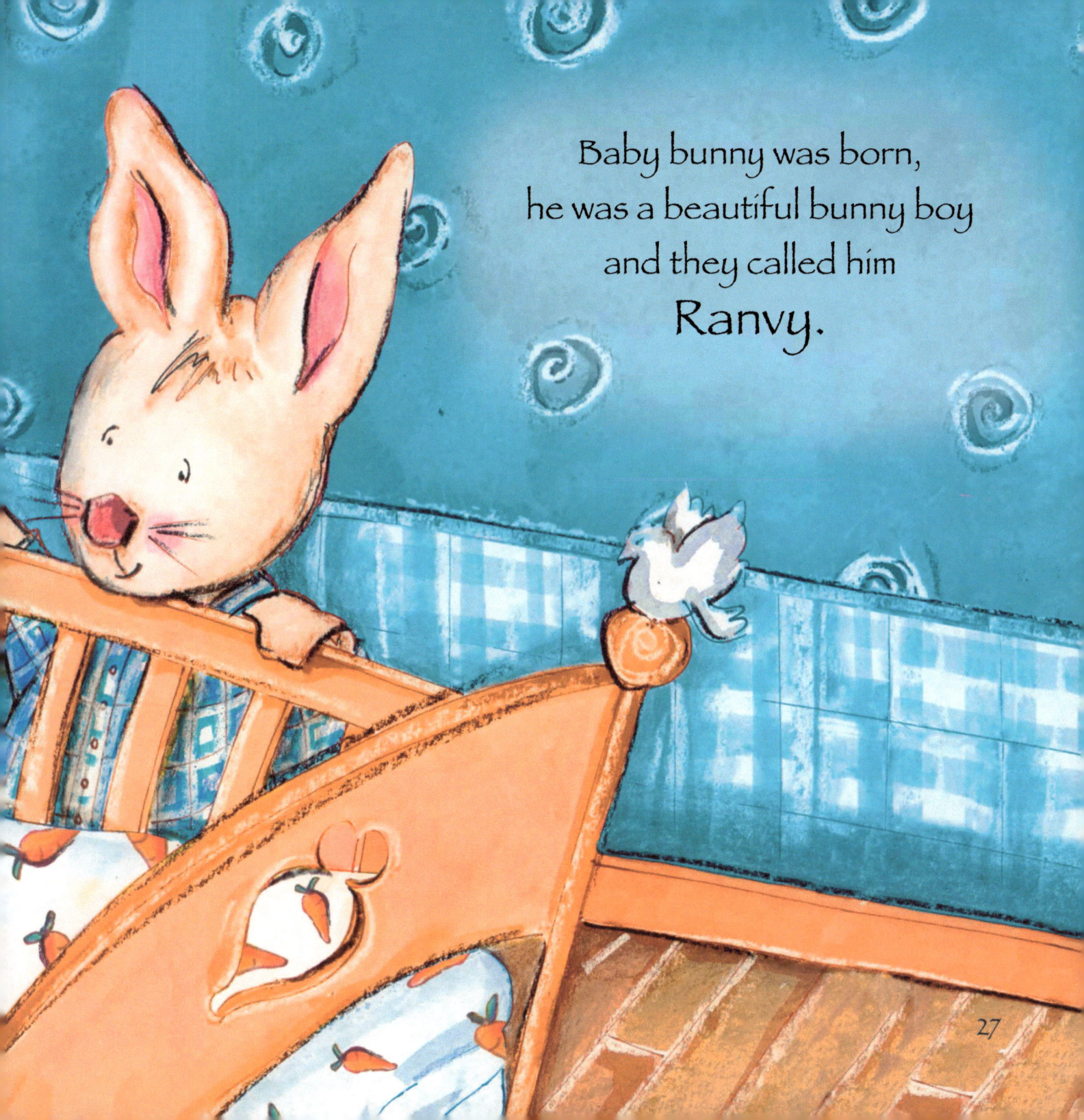

Baby bunny was born,
he was a beautiful bunny boy
and they called him
Ranvy.

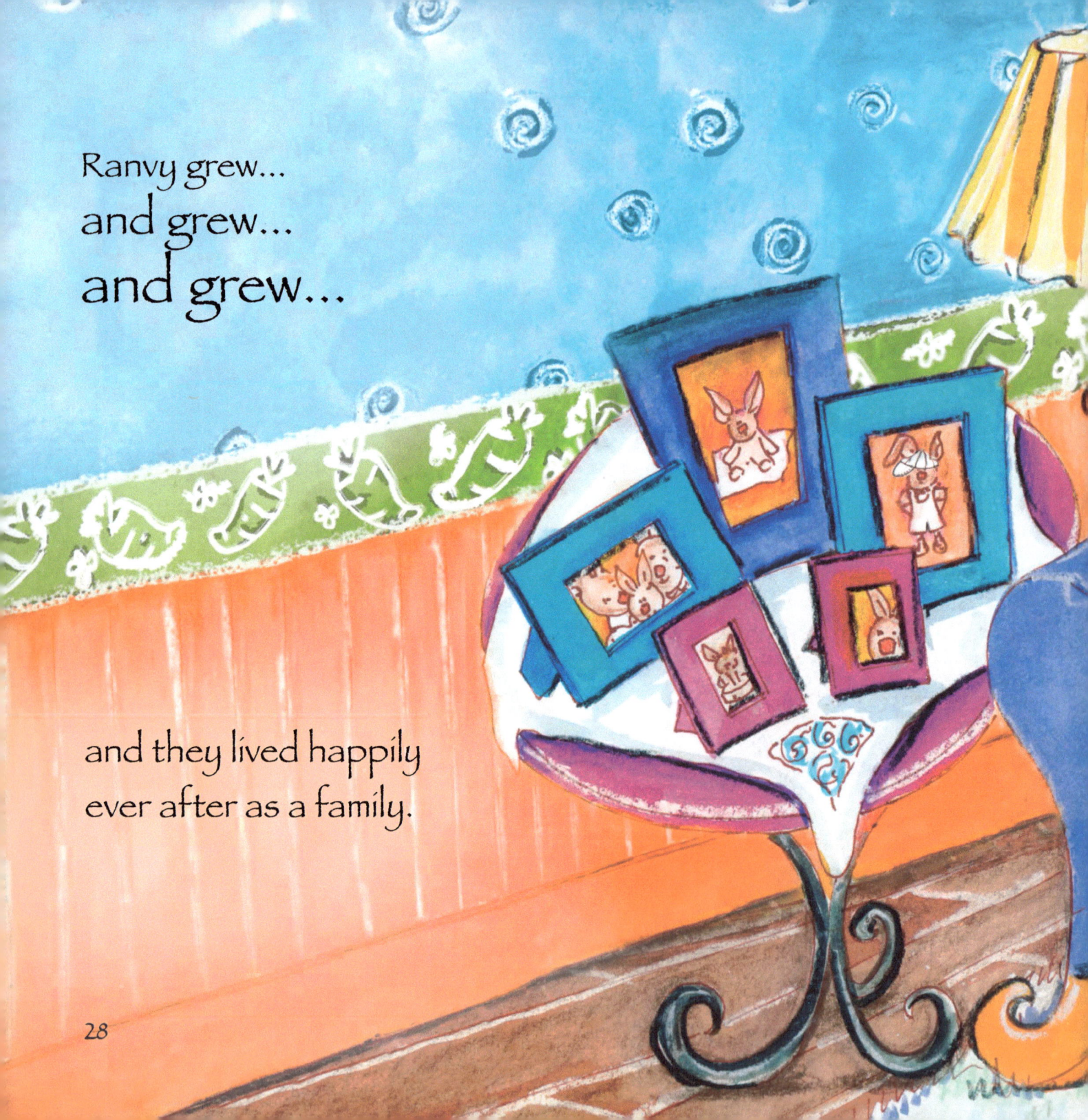

Ranvy grew...
 and grew...
  and grew...

and they lived happily ever after as a family.

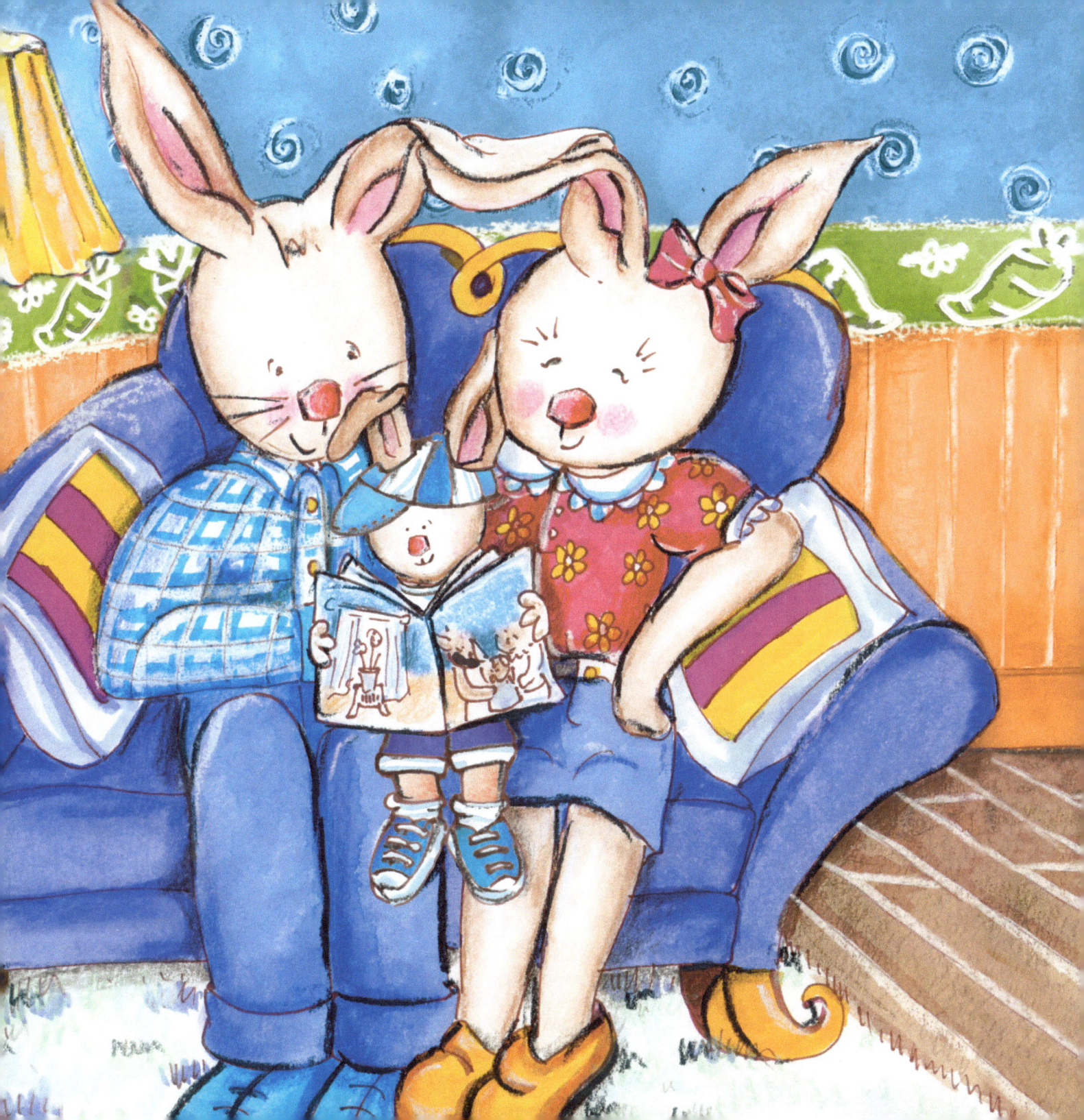

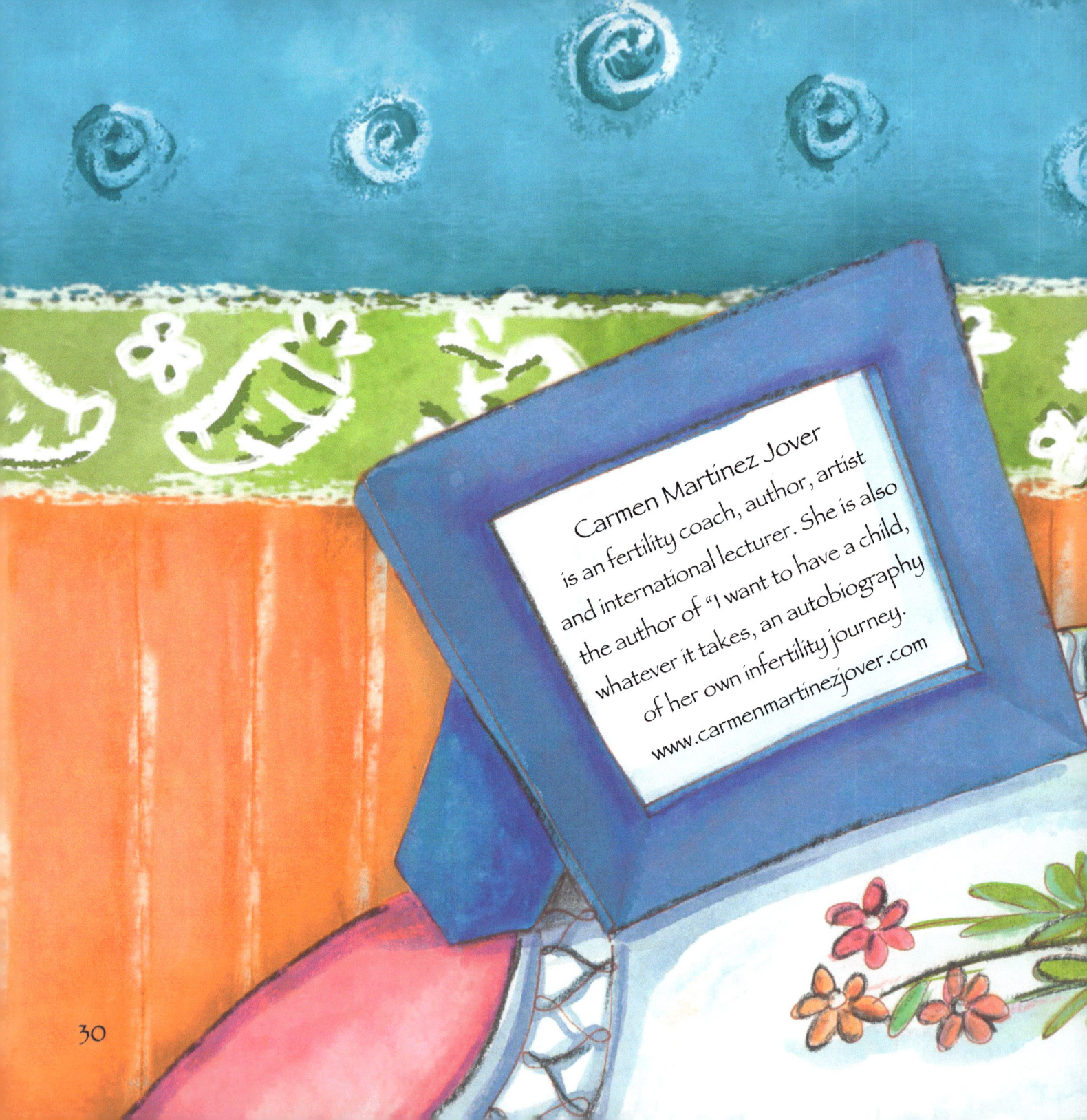

Carmen Martinez Jover is an fertility coach, author, artist and international lecturer. She is also the author of "I want to have a child, whatever it takes, an autobiography of her own infertility journey.
www.carmenmartinezjover.com

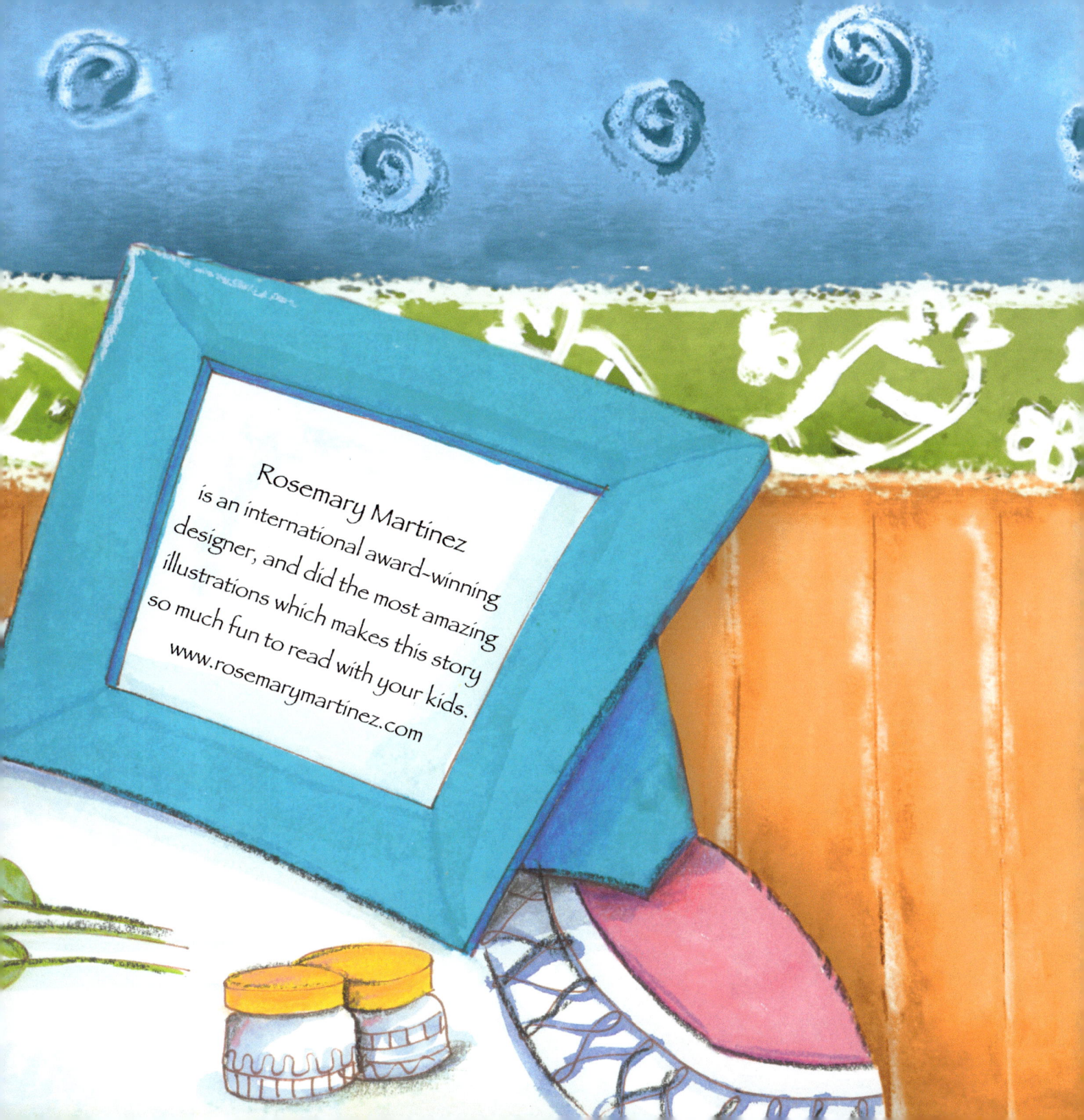

Rosemary Martinez is an international award-winning designer, and did the most amazing illustrations which makes this story so much fun to read with your kids.
www.rosemarymartinez.com

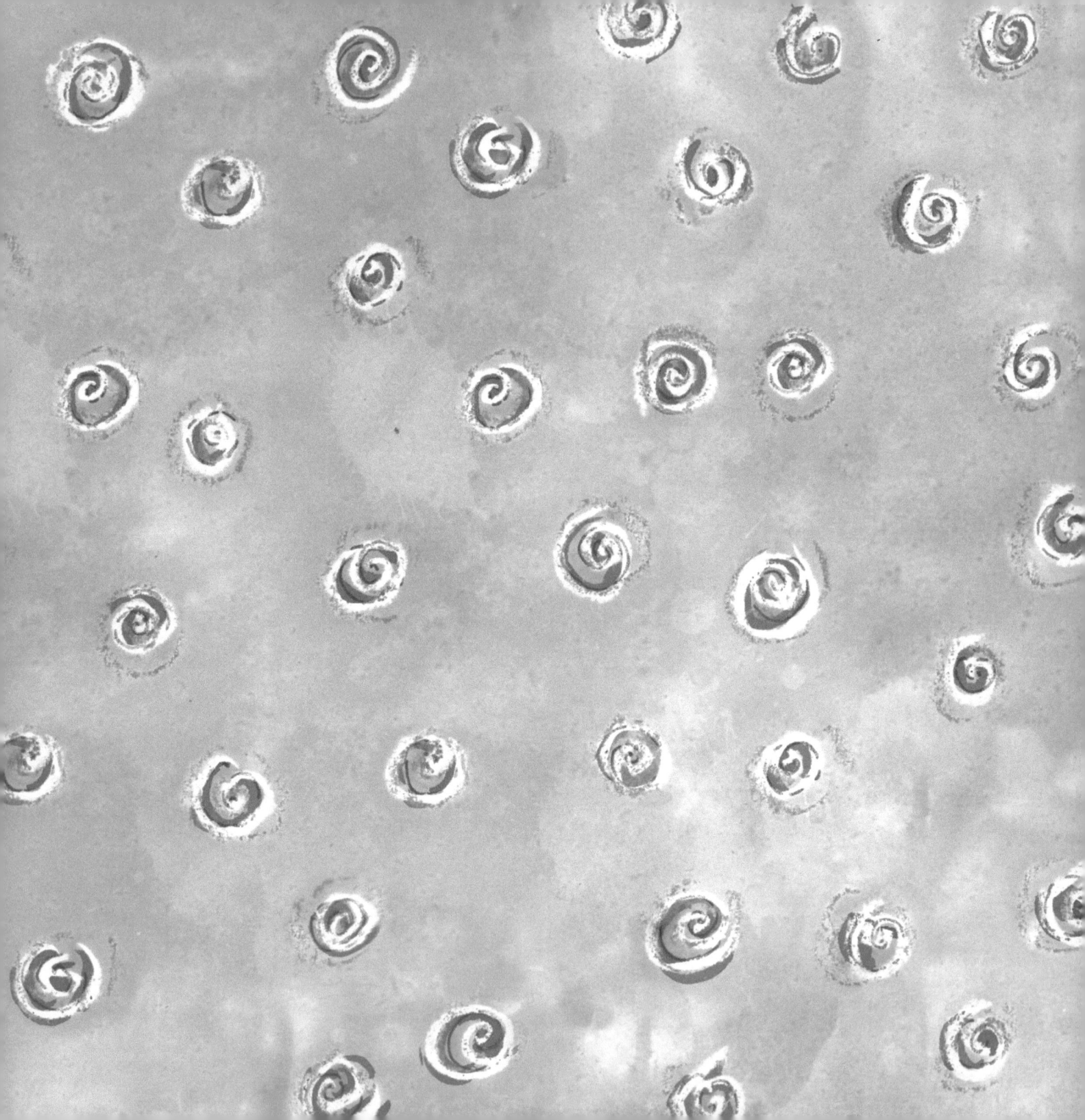

Be the heroes of your own story

Personalise your own story with your own names

https://books.carmenmartinezjover.com

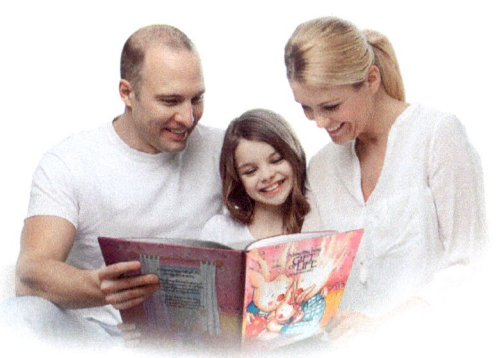

EGG DONATION

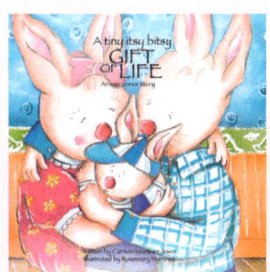 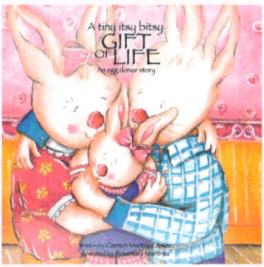 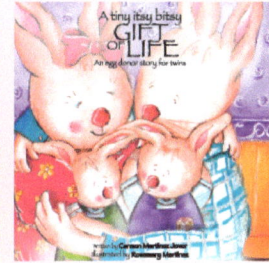

A tiny itsy bitsy gift of life, an egg donor story for girls, boys and twins. **PERSONALISED**

ADOPTION

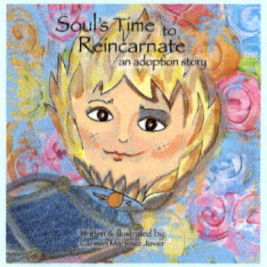

Soul's Time to Reincarnate, an adoption story. **PERSONALISED**

SINGLE MUM BY CHOICE

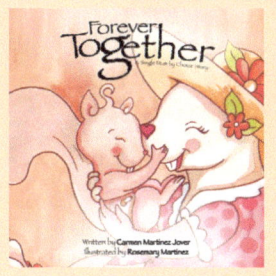 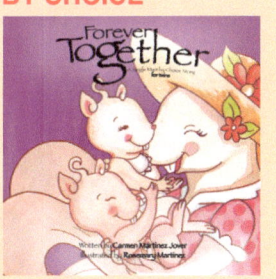

Forever Together, a single mum by choice story for one child or twins. **PERSONALISED**

TWO DADS

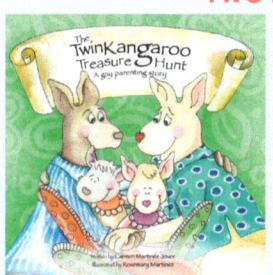 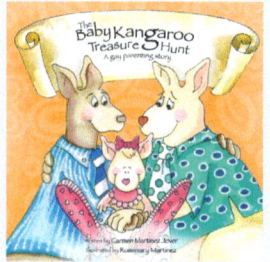

The baby kangaroo treasure hunt, a gay parenting story for one child or twins. **PERSONALISED**

Other books by: Carmen Martinez Jover

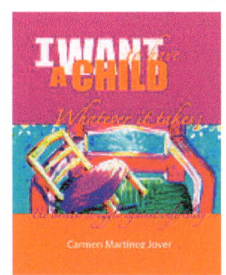 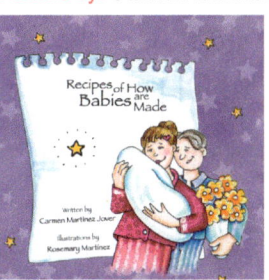 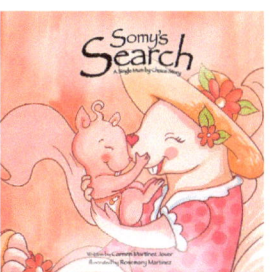

I want to have a child, whatever it takes!

Recipes of How Babies are Made

Somy's Search, a single mum by choice story

Available in:

www.amazon.com
www.carmenmartinezjover.com

English, Español, Français, Italiano, Português, Svenska, Русский, Nederlands

www.ingramcontent.com/pod-product-compliance
Lightning Source LLC
Chambersburg PA
CBHW042020080426

42735CB00002B/116